Every Body's Fitness Book

Every Body's Fitness Book

A Simple, Safe, and Sane Approach to Personal Fitness

by GORDON W. STEWART, M.Sc.

Illustrated by Jack Crane

A Dolphin Book
Doubleday & Company, Inc., Garden City, New York   1980
Doubleday Canada, Ltd., Toronto

Acknowledgment

I favor private thank-yous over public listings. Many friends, all professionals in their own special fields, offered valued advice toward the preparation of this book. Their assistance will always be remembered.

The 12-Minute Walking/Running Test, The 12-Minute Cycling Test, The 3-Mile Walking Test, and The 12-Minute Swimming Test are from *The Aerobics Way* by Kenneth H. Cooper, M.D., M.P.H. Copyright © 1977 by Kenneth H. Cooper. Reprinted by permission of the publisher, M. Evans and Company, Inc., New York, New York 10017.

Library of Congress Cataloging in Publication Data Stewart, Gordon W Every body's fitness book. (A Dolphin book) 1. Physical fitness. 2. Exercise. I. Title. RA781.S85 613.7 ISBN: 0-385-15199-3 Library of Congress Catalog Card Number 79–7219 Copyright © 1980 by Gordon W. Stewart All Rights Reserved Printed in the United States of America First Edition

Dedicated to

Dr. Bill Ross
my teacher, colleague, and fine friend
and to
the Out-to-lunch Bunch
and the Dusty Sneakers
who taught me as much as I taught them.

Contents

Preface

As a teacher of fitness, I spend much time rescuing people in a sea of confusion. This book is, in part, a response to that confusion. It intends to answer the questions most commonly asked and simplify the issues most often misunderstood. I propose to do this, not by directly confronting these questions and issues, not by wading through the controversy; instead, by wiping the slate clean and starting again. This means going back to the basics and considering the proper principles of exercise. There aren't that many of them and the logic behind them isn't that difficult to grasp. But they're crucial. They serve as the foundation for all fitness activities.

Donald Pruden, in *Around Town Cycling*, said, "One of the beauties of teaching is that the teacher often learns as much as he imparts." With experience, he also learns *how much* to impart. This is important in an age of fitness overeducation where information seems overlapping and sometimes contradictory. There's an important difference between what is necessary and what is merely interesting. You need the basics to start. Details can wait. Entire books have been written on various activities, but this is a starter book and, try as I might, I just couldn't think of anything else that *needed* to be included.

As a book for beginners, *Every Body's Fitness Book* aims to avoid the shortcomings of some of its predecessors. Many books in the field follow a recipe, "test tube," do-this-and-you-get-this approach. That's fine in the laboratory and works well with rats but it's not that simple out in the world of people. There may be injuries, setbacks, and boredom, but much joy. These issues must be dealt with. I have spent a number of years in the "trenches," so to speak, helping adults of all sizes, shapes, dispositions, interests, and aptitudes reclaim their bodies and move down the road to fitness. I have watched their trials and tribulations and, in this book, rely heavily on what I learned from them. These are the practical and "people" parts of fitness and very important as they take it beyond the "test tube" stage.

A second kind of book, those dealing only with one activity, charts a narrow path. Based on the assumption that theirs is the activity for you, they go about telling you how to pursue it. Books on running are, at present, most abundant. This book is a sidestep, out from behind all the running information. Making no assumptions, it helps with one of the most important decisions facing beginners—picking the activity that's best for you. Tastes and interests vary. Each person must find his own appropriate medium for physical expression if habitual, lifelong activity is to result. If you're absolutely and utterly convinced you're not a runner, then, for heaven's sake, don't go out and run to get fit.

A few books impart misinformation. Books on exercises are often the worst offenders. Some include exercises that just aren't meant to be, dangerous for the less fit and relatively inactive, and inappropriate for even the healthiest of people. Some authors rely heavily on personal bias. This is unfortunate. There is no place for personal bias in books advising *others* about *their* health and fitness.

Some fascinating books talk of the spirit of movement, the joy and exhilaration that is physical activity after fitness. Few books on fitness even hint of these feelings, this other state, and, hence miss one of the most important reasons to work through the time of commitment and perseverance that is the early part of any reconditioning program. As Colin Fletcher says in *The New Complete Walker*, we mustn't let the "ways and means" mask the "joys and insights" physical activity can bring. To talk only of how to do it and how good it is for you, and not how good it feels, somehow cheapens physical activity.

So this book aims to help those returning to fitness after months, years (or even decades!) of inactivity, those who have tried and failed and those who are persevering, not content with their activity and, perhaps, looking for something new. Some of the finer technical points can even help the happily active facing periodic setbacks or problems with their routine. And last, it's for teachers, in the hopes they'll be sensitive in leading others to improved personal health and fitness.

It takes the following approach:

- It doesn't humor or mislead. Achieving fitness is not easy, but neither should you make it hard on yourself.
- It strives for technical accuracy. If readers are to be educated, then proper education is paramount.
- It details a smorgasbord of activities. Great pains are taken to help *you* find what's right for *you*.
- It couples the practical and the philosophical. The "how to" information is really only a means to an end. It hopes to get you through the door of fitness to those good feelings that come a few months and a few miles down the road.

You'll soon find that there are three of me at work here. My professional self, the teacher in me, offers the "how to" advice. It's to help you through the early part when steps are slow and, at times, unsteady. My practical self talks of how good being active makes you feel. If you stay with it, you'll soon understand what he's going on about. But my personal self says there's more to it than this. He says the other two are missing the most important part—the good feeling that comes *after* fitness. The "after fitness" part is what many seem to be talking about these days. And no wonder. It's the best part of all.

Gord Stewart
October 1978

How to Read It, How to Use It

As a how-to book, *Every Body's Fitness Book* is meant to be read *and* used. There is great hope from this end that it will become your friendly companion and guide—a teacher in your pocket—tattered and worn from use, not crisp and fresh on the shelf after a single reading.

You might follow its advice alone. Or it might guide you and family or friends along your chosen road to fitness. Or if you, too, are a teacher of fitness, it can help you bring an informal and individualized approach to group activities.

It follows the "verdict now, evidence later" approach, taking this tack for two main reasons. First, the importance of activity is understood and accepted. No need to belabor the point. Second, I've learned there isn't a great deal *I* can do to convince *anyone* they should start. You only start when you're good and ready. But once you've made that decision, I can help. And that's what this book intends to do. I'll tell you *how* to start now, and later on get back to the issue of *why* you should start.

Following the introductory chapter, Chapters Two and Three are the foundation for the remainder of the book. Chapter Two sets out the Five Steps to Fitness:

> STEP ONE: A health checklist for pre-activity clearance and some testing information.
> STEP TWO: Pre-activity planning.
> STEP THREE: Precautions and special advice.
> STEP FOUR: The game plan for fitness—the FITTness Formula—and some tips for teachers.
> STEP FIVE: Principles for Persisting.

Chapter Three, "The Stretch Bit," offers suppleness and strength exercises. There is no attempt to convince you they're fun, although, if you take your time, you'll soon find them pleasurable and relaxing. And they are *very* important, for the reasons soon to be mentioned. Only sensible and conservative exercises that can be adequately portrayed by word and picture have been included.

Chapters Four through Eight build on this base, giving the specifics of walking, running, cycling, swimming, and indoor activities. I catalogue these activities because there are many ways to fitness, and what's appealing to one may be quite uninteresting to another. This book aims to help you decide what's right for you, remembering that what's right now may not always be. Your tastes and interests may change with time or changing seasons, and unforeseen setbacks may alter your plans. Snow may force you out of your regular routine to an indoor maintenance program. If you overdo it as a runner or cyclist, the swimming chapter may sometime prove useful.

You'll get tips on proper progression; how to start and how to keep going; common injuries and how to avoid them; clothing, equipment, and supplies.

View the Chapter Two injuries advice with some detachment. It's an after-the-fact discussion of what to do *if* you get hurt. Don't dwell on it now. Return to it later if the need arises. More important, spend time with the injury-prevention information in specific-activity chapters. Attention paid there can mean less need to refer back to the Chapter Two "fix up" advice later on.

Clothing and equipment advice is important. Proper equipment selection ensures comfort, less risk of injury, and greater enjoyment from your activity—factors that greatly affect your chance of success. Moreover, this advice can help you discern necessity from accessory in the event you come across a salesperson who is less than sympathetic to *your* needs.

Talk of prices is pointless because of their relentless march upward. Instead, discussion focuses on qualities and characteristics you should look for. You'll soon discover what you must pay to get the quality you're after.

The structure of each chapter is determined largely by the information to be conveyed. Of necessity, some chapters are considerably longer than others. There's more to buying a bike than there is to buying a bathing suit.

To help you when your interest grows, there's a short and select reading list at the end of each chapter.

The outdoor people may find Chapter Nine disheartening. Space devoted to their activities is not to suggest that they are less important than the others, just less accessible. The fitness principles still apply, but, to avoid being encyclopedic, I refer you to the various experts for specific advice.

Guide books are not necessarily designed for cover-to-cover reading. Pick out that information that proves useful to you now. Why labor over running-shoe advice if you're ready to head for the pool?

If you're anxious to get started, read Chapters One, Two, and Three carefully. Next go to the activity of your choice. Proceed to Chapters Nine, Ten, and Eleven; then, if you wish, double back to the chapters you bypassed earlier. They should serve as general-interest and future-reference material.

Remember, in this quest for fitness, not to lose sight of the total picture. Good health should be the goal, and sufficient fitness is only one aspect of positive health. Other lifestyle habits deserve strong consideration. Regular physical activity is important, but proper dietary habits and a sensible approach to smoking and drinking are of equal importance. In fact, if you're in the market for lifestyle change and are a very heavy smoker, you'd be wise to strive for nonsmoking status first and move on to fitness later. If you're after weight loss, dietary-change and physical-activity programs work well together. Other than this, go for one change at a time. Start winning in one area, then move on to your next task. A series of small sucesses add up to one large victory. How many New Year's resolutions to "stop smoking, drink less, lose weight, and get active" have you heard proclaimed? How many succeeded?

Finally, plan to be patient. Fitness, like anything of great consequence, is not easily or quickly won. Look for results over the long term, not overnight. Don't rush or force fitness. Push too hard and the body rebels, but treat it sensibly and with respect and it will perform remarkably.

Whatever you can do, or dream you can, begin it.
Boldness has genius, power, and magic in it.

—Goethe

CHAPTER ONE

Fence Mending

AN INTRODUCTION

November 5. It was a red-letter day for abuse to fitness nuts.

I stood at the top of "my hill" in the classic postrace runner's pose. Hunched over, hands on knees, legs wobbly, and heart pounding, I breathed deeply and quickly.

An elderly lady, who had been watching me curiously, approached.

"You really shouldn't do that, you know!"

"Oh, really," I gasped. "Why not?"

"Because it destroys the natural rhythm of your heart."

"It speeds it up, doesn't it?" I retaliated.

"That's right!" She smiled with obvious satisfaction.

"Oh well, it'll slow down again in a minute or two," I said and headed abruptly down the hill in preparation for another charge to the top.

I guess I should have stopped to talk to her. I could have explained that as an athlete I am prepared for and require this demanding, maximum kind of activity. But she was on the right track. You don't have to be an athlete to be fit, and for adults striving for basic fitness, the routine I demonstrated is unnecessary and, in some cases, undesirable. But she was the third intrusion on my world and "my hill" that day, and my patience had run out so I just carried on my way.

This hill I refer to really isn't mine. The city owns it, but I know it well, so I lay claim to it. It has two parts. Two stop lights cover 400 yards, and once you learn the system it's green lights all the way. The first part isn't steep, just enough to let you know you're going uphill. The top half of the hill (from the hydrant to the little tree) offers 190 yards of sidewalk snaking uphill, so you can't see where you finish until you're almost there. Perhaps this is just as well. In weaker moments, you can fantasize that the end is near.

Along with its steep slope and twisting turns, this hill has somewhat of a local reputation. Known as "Cardiac Crest," it's the most direct route between the local YMCA and a big, beautiful park bordering the ocean. The "Y" beginners have been taught well. Wisely, they detour one block east and pursue a more gentle path to the park.

"Cardiac Crest" has wide sidewalks, and the motorists are generally friendly. It's an excellent place for a runner to prepare for the coming season. There's speed and strength in those hills and, if you spend enough time with them, a measure of it rubs off.

On a good day I can cover the 190-yard top half of the hill in about 28 seconds. On other days, 32 seconds seem more appropriate.

This day the motorists were not so friendly. About halfway up the hill on my first run I sensed a car off my left shoulder climbing no faster than I. It crept on, pulling even, then finally edged in front. I looked straight ahead, then curiosity got the better of me and I glanced left. A young couple, riding comfortably, gazed at me in disbelief. I smiled and flashed the peace sign. They smiled and drove on, apparently satisfied. I was alone to finish the hill.

A few minutes later as I jogged slowly downhill a carload of teen-agers passed. In unison and with little originality they yelled, "Faster." I greeted them with a not-so-friendly sign and they, too, carried on their way laughing and yelling, victorious, perhaps in search of another victim. Alone again, I wondered what I had done to deserve this.

These stares, yells, and the lecture made me wonder if we had somehow slipped back in time. Nowadays fitness nuts can go through their routine in relative anonymity. Honking horns and ridicule are pretty much things of the past. Over the past decade there's been an increased awareness of the importance of activity. Friends and neighbors who aren't active leave us "movers" alone. Perhaps it's a tinge of guilt. If they aren't joining us, they really know they should be.

We may be winning our neighbors over, but their dogs certainly aren't catching on. Their attitude is historically unchanged. The few abusive ones make us wary of them all.

A recent run brought me the dogs and with them some other irritations. I got a bug in my eye, my socks kept falling down, and my legs were itchy. Nevertheless, it was an exceptionally fragrant early-spring day. The city skyline and ocean beaches were unusually clear and beautiful. I seemed to flow along lightly, effortlessly as I ran. I looked forward to the challenge of the coming hills. My body moved naturally and comfortably without guidance. My mind was free to ponder other matters, my eyes to capture the passing scene and my senses to fully experience the beginnings of spring.

But the biggest memory is the dogs. Some came alone, others in pairs. I encountered thirteen in all—a personal record. Seeking adventure, I toured residential streets, ran down alleys and along paths that until then I didn't know existed. The dogs were lying in ambush.

A Doberman pinscher and a German shepherd, a terrifying pair, met me first. I made a meek and narrow escape. The next encounters were with a small dog (who I assume was the front man) and a big black dog who looked like a wolf.

A Samoyed was the first four-legged creature I encountered who left me alone. Perhaps jogger chasing is a demeaning activity in the Samoyed world. I was sufficiently paranoid near the end of my run to detour a toy poodle lounging on the sidewalk in front of his house. This must have done his ego a world of good. Eight antagonists out of thirteen—not at all a good average.

Objectionable people and irreverent dogs can be disconcerting to the beginner. But you grow immune to them and soon they are quickly forgotten annoyances. However, inappropriate exercise classes, fitness "fiction," and previous bad experiences prove more troublesome. For these are the roots of confusion.

Exercise classes that insist upon the principles of athletic training guarantee injuries and bad publicity. "Dropouts" will tell their friends that getting fit is a most difficult task and perhaps not worth the effort. The fit survive, and those who need it most may be spectators once again. Pain, torture, and agony are counterproductive and leave an exercise leader with a small core of participants who really don't need his guidance. They're already there. Physiotherapists, sports-medicine types, and orthopedic surgeons are busy tending to those who tried for too much too soon.

A classic villain is the preski class. It's disheartening when a young friend returns from her second class saying, "Last week the gym was packed. You couldn't even move. Was I ever stiff and sore the next day. But it's O.K. now. I feel better and there were only half as many tonight so we had lots of room." There's a natural attrition rate in most exercise classes since some recruits are not prepared for the modest effort and dedication necessary in the early stages. It's disappointing, though, when attrition is partially due to an instructor's insensitivity to the needs and abilities of those in his class.

Some exercise alone and inflict this same approach on themselves. Perhaps a previous teacher advised to bounce, jerk, and strain their way to fitness. Their chance of success is reduced, their risk of injury increased if they choose this route. And what of the innocent bystander who may be contemplating a move to fitness himself? Our straining friend is, at best, a bad example.

Fitness "fiction" is equally bothersome. There's general agreement that—regardless of age and level of fitness—vigorous activities can be pursued and satisfying improvements can be expected if one progresses patiently and sensibly. I once came across an article that took a different approach. It was aimed at the middle-aged and older group and it implied: "Take it easy, don't exert yourself, or you're asking for trouble." It was a gathering of misinformation, half truths, and scare tactics about exercise, but I knew I was in for trouble.

We were into the third week of our spring exercise classes. Our beginners were on their way. Slowly and surely it was getting easier. They said it felt nice to be moving again. But for those who read the article, conflicting information had met them in midstream and they were confused.

One man, who had been sufficiently educated, kidded, "I'm over forty, I guess I should be in a wheelchair." Two ladies didn't take it so lightly. For one, this was her last class. She and her husband had both read the article and decided she shouldn't be jogging. The other departed shortly after with similar sentiments. She had been convinced that "Brisk walking is fine, but jogging isn't good for anyone."

Some magazine articles err on the other side. One detailed a three-month marathon training program suggesting you can run twenty-six miles three months hence if you're a daily half-hour runner now. If anyone asked me about it, I urged, "Do each week's program three times before moving on. That'll give you a nine-month buildup. And be careful. Even that might be too fast." I figured that four out of five who insisted on following this accelerated program would be injured in the process and wouldn't make their deadline. Unfortunately, at last count, my estimates proved fairly accurate.

The issue is further confused when fact is built on fiction. An article in our local newspaper extolled the virtues of a sawdust running trail newly installed in a city park. In praising the advantages of the soft surface, the writer implied that no one should risk running one step on a sidewalk or road.

I telephoned her to voice my concern. I pointed out that if you progress gradually, have proper running style, and wear shoes that adequately support the feet, then sidewalks and roads present no dangers. Now *she* knew, but the damage was already done.

Moving on to the bookstore, further confusion awaits. When I go, I usually head straight for the "Health . . . Beauty . . . Fitness" section or whatever title is given to those books that guide us to better bodies and calmer minds. I always find the odd book suggesting exercises that just aren't meant to be—ones that make physiotherapists cringe and shake their heads. In their own quiet way, these books may cause some well-intentioned people to join the ranks of the walking wounded.

Misinformed writers are a minority but some are able to sneak a few words into the popular press. This may result because many academics spend their time writing for professional journals when really they should be filtering more hard facts down to the popular publications.

Facts are needed to counter the fiction provided by some who are not as well trained but more prolific. It's this fiction that causes a twenty-year-old to say, "Older people shouldn't jog, they'll have heart attacks," and a forty-five-year-old architect to ask about a marathoner his age, "Is it possible he won't live as long?"

But the greatest confusion may come from previous bad experiences. It's a difficult task to convince someone that physical activity can be painless, positive, and even personally meaningful if, in their school, running was used for punishment or slower running meant lower grades. Those who were overweight, slow, and unco-ordinated in their youth or those who got "two laps and twenty-five pushups" if they were late for gym class have much to forget before they can set off peacefully toward fitness.

Ah, but I promised not to dwell on the confusion. Let's go back to the beginning. Good health is what we're after. Robert Frost once said, "Good fences make good neighbors." Well, good habits bring good health.

In 1972, *Preventive Medicine* journal reported a five-year study of seven thousand adults showing that seven simple habits were associated with longer life and better health. The habits:

- Three meals a day at regular intervals.
- Eating breakfast.
- Moderate exercise.
- Seven to eight hours' sleep nightly.
- Moderate weight.
- No smoking.
- Alcohol in moderation or not at all.

If you choose the right activities, the moderate-exercise habit leads to fitness. Fitness, quite simply, has three important components. Call them the three s's—stamina, suppleness, and strength. Oh, athletes need more. They train long hours and along with the three s's come balance, co-ordination, agility, and speed. Children are more fortunate. They come by their fitness quite naturally. Dawn-to-dusk nonstop movement—climbing trees and playing tag —ensures them of bodies that move with ease and efficiency. But for adults returning to fitness, the basic three s's are quite enough.

Stamina is one's distance from fatigue. It's a simple word meaning the same as cardiovascular or cardiorespiratory endurance. It has to do with how easily the lungs take in oxygen and how efficiently the heart pumps the oxygen-rich blood around to the various body parts and internal organs. Sufficient stamina means you tire less quickly and it seems to reduce the risk of coronary heart disease.

Suppleness (alias flexibility) plays its part in maintaining proper posture, reducing stiffness and soreness from unaccustomed activity, and minimizing the risk of low-back problems.

The *strength* you're after isn't the "big bicep, kick-sand-in-the-face" variety. It's merely sufficient strength of the stomach muscles (to minimize undue strain on the muscles of the lower back) and enough overall body strength to allow normal daily tasks to be accomplished with ease and comfort.

In fairness to the issue, and to keep the nutritionists happy, our three s's should be expanded to include the additional important factor of weight control. You can possess great stamina, suppleness, and strength, but you're not totally fit if overweight. Sufficient physical activity helps balance the caloric bank. If intake (by eating) and expenditure (through daily activity) don't balance, a "debit" or a "credit" ensues. Unfortunately, "credit" is most common and manifests itself in excess and unwanted fat.

Stamina, suppleness, strength, and weight control—three s's and a w? *This* is fitness, and the President's Council on Physical Fitness and Sports says it brings:

> the ability to carry out daily tasks with vigor and alertness, without undue fatigue, and with ample energy to enjoy leisure-time pursuits and to meet unforeseen emergencies.

Achieving basic fitness and maintaining it is a noble and worthy goal. But there's more to it than this, and I'd fail if I ended the discussion here. I'm an habitual, addicted "mover," and I know that fitness is really only a stopping-off point between inactivity and something more. As a teacher I've come to learn that those who want only quick, tangible results don't often last. But those who progress slowly, those who keep an open mind and can contemplate the intangible, are soon rewarded. The "ways and means" get you to fitness. The "joys and insights" are the rewards that come after.

These rewards are, at once, unique, volatile, deeply meaningful, and almost impossible to explain to others. They're *feelings* and they take you from the stage of wanting to exercise to the point where you really can't go without it.

You can start by breaking free from a world of elevators, cars and televisions—a world that calls out, "Relax. Take it easy." If you persist and find the right activity, it's soon relaxing and invigorating. It becomes a daily looked-forward-to routine, a chunk of freedom in a busy day (not to mention a socially acceptable means of escape!). You may soon find yourself going to great and devious means to protect your sacred hour in the pool or out on the road.

But still, it's more than this. Some days are special, both exhilarating and joyous. Howard Mickel says:

> I enjoy the very feel of my body and its rhythms, the production of sweat, and the love affair that developed between myself and Kansas skies, country roads, grass, ponds, and winds.

Dr. George Sheehan suggests that these powerful feelings await us all.

For every runner who tours the world running marathons, there are thousands who run to hear the leaves and listen to the rain and look to the day when it all is suddenly as easy as a bird in flight. For them sport is not a test but a therapy, not a trial but a reward, not a question but an answer.

But, for now, we must go back to the basics. Chapters Two and Three give advice to get you safely through the fitness part. This is of utmost importance. Unless fitness is achieved, the rest remains pure speculation.

CHAPTER TWO

Starting and Persisting

FIVE STEPS TO FITNESS

STEP ONE: THE HEALTH CHECKLIST—
PRE-ACTIVITY CLEARANCE

STEP TWO: PLANNING
Time of Day, The Hassle Factor,
Class Searching, Activity Choosing

STEP THREE: PRECAUTIONS
Special Cases, Weight Loss, Smoking,
Drinking, Pitfalls, Warning Signs,
Warmup and Cooldown

STEP FOUR: THE FITTNESS FORMULA
Frequency (How Often?),
Intensity (How Hard?),
Time (How Long?),
Type (What Activity?)

STEP FIVE: PRINCIPLES FOR PERSISTING
Patience, Weight Loss or Not,
Don't Rush, Record Your Workouts,
Boredom, Injuries, Rewards,
The Right Activity

Special Tips for Teachers

MY SIDELINE view offered a new perspective. Watching a friend teach a class, I was unencumbered by the specifics of teaching and clear to see the overall scheme of things. For the first time I really understood how difficult it is to start—how important are the first few steps.

Before me was a class of middle-aged men and women *learning to run*. No doubt they moved with ease in their childhood but something had been lost in the interim. Now they were starting to move again. They were led through a gentle warmup. Explanations were neatly tucked between exercises, a subtle way of offering much-needed rest. Following the large group warmup, a few veterans headed out into the crisp fall for small group or solo runs. The newcomers remained inside. Soft trails and grassy fields must wait for later. Under a watchful eye, they were assured a leisurely beginning. If they heeded advice, their chance of making it to the trails and fields was excellent.

This was a most significant moment. If only they knew what lay ahead. For now, running wouldn't be totally easy and carefree. But a few months and a few miles away, things could be different.

My run of the previous evening was on my mind as I watched this class. I know it was these lingering feelings of yesterday that made me so sensitive to the fascination that awaited them.

It had been one of those eastern fall days that time and the West tug from the memory. The evening air was a reminder that, along with its unmatched color, fall is very much a transition from breezy summer to the harsh reality of winter.

A friend advised, "Run down along the canal. It's a mile between bridges." I headed south from downtown. The canal was calm and the adjoining green belt ensured a quiet time. Walkers and cyclists were out in full force, along with an extraordinary number of runners.

I ran by elegant homes, got a glimpse of the university across the way, and passed a football practice where forty-yard dashes and stadium stairs were the orders of the day. I wished for them a slow run by the canal.

I left my watch at the hotel, choosing my friend's bridges as my guide. In my exuberance to explore new territory, I must have lost count of the bridges. The reward for my mistake was a sunset and a run back to the lights of downtown in darkness. My beer and dinner tasted exceptionally fine that evening.

So I thought of that run as I watched this class, and I was pulling for them. I hoped they would persist and one day run by that canal. Time and patience were needed. Great things lay ahead.

The advice in this chapter aims to get *you* started sensibly and help *you* persist. Let it guide you as you progress. Combine it with the Chapter Three exercises and the chapter outlining the activity of your choice. Refer to it regularly. Return to it for moral support at times when you wonder if it's worth the effort, and remember: "It don't come easy."

In the information that follows, I won't offer points to win, suggest a "daily dozen" to be done during TV commercials, or prescribe distances to cover in specified times. (I'm not offering a system for you to adapt to.) Instead, I suggest a more leisurely and informal approach. The following guidelines are to help you make up your own system. I merely say, "Start moving!" Peruse the activities of Chapters Four through Nine. Choose something that can offer *you* a measure of enjoyment and satisfaction from the very beginning (while remembering that something else may prove better later).

A "daily dozen" and other regimented routines no doubt bring fitness. But if you aim only for fitness you may fall short of the target. If you choose the right activity, you stand a better chance of winning fitness and you might even capture some of the good things that come after—the fascination that Howard Mickel and George Sheehan speak of.

The advice to get you started toward these fascinations comes in five parts. Step One is the Health Checklist—Pre-Activity Clearance. Step Two involves some thoughtful planning. You have four decisions to make before you face your first day of action. Step Three encompasses the final preparation, offering seven precautions you should consider. Step Four is the game plan for starting. Four factors make up the FITTness Formula. Once started, you must look to the long term. Step Five outlines some Principles for Persisting.

Step One
The Health Checklist—Pre-Activity Clearance

Some start right in. Others feel, or a professional suggests, that they should begin with some sort of test. A wide assortment of tests can measure your stamina, suppleness, and strength. The stamina tests range from simple and inexpensive to time-consuming and costly.

Two types of stamina tests exist. One is a diagnostic test that we'll call an *exercise-tolerance test*. These are administered by health professionals and are available in a variety of settings, including hospitals, many doctors' offices, and some fitness centers. Some tests are conducted on a stationary exercise bike designed for testing (called a bicycle ergometer). Others are done on a larger and more expensive piece of apparatus called a treadmill. In either case, the subject being tested is connected via electrodes and wires to a machine called an electrocardiogram. The electrocardiogram monitors the activity of the heart, recording irregularities in heart function and, thereby, assists in diagnosing the existence and extent of coronary artery disease. The more sophisticated the diagnostic test, the greater the cost.

The second kind of test, which we'll term a *fitness test*, is an estimator. Medical diagnosis is not involved; the test merely estimates your fitness. The speed of the heart rate after a prescribed amount of work (a timed walk-run, or a step test, for example) indicates fitness level. Fitness tests are easier to administer and available in most fitness and recreation centers and YMCAs and YWCAs. Some are designed for self-administration, two of which will be discussed shortly. Many programs use a beginning fitness test for motivation and as a bench mark to chart improvement.

A "test" or "not test" controversy centers around whether an exercise-tolerance test should precede an exercise program. The pro-test group calls it a "wise precaution," the antitest group says it's an "unnecessary obstacle." An interesting outcome of *most* positive exercise-tolerance tests is the recommendation to embark on *gradual and progressive exercise*—exactly what is being suggested here anyway. Per-Olaf Åstrand, the famous Swedish physiologist, once made an interesting comment on exercise-tolerance tests. He suggested that, in the light of the increasing evidence of the benefits of physical activity, those choosing to remain inactive should be the ones tested to see if they can afford that kind of lifestyle.

Fortunately, there is a path of least resistance. This path includes the use of a handy, self-administered questionnaire known as PAR-Q—the Physical Activity Readiness Questionnaire. The concept of this questionnaire was developed by a panel of professionals, then researched and designed by the Ministry of Health in the province of British Columbia. The questionnaire's main purpose is to act as a first-level screening device. It aids in identifying the small number of adults for whom physical activity is inappropriate or those who should have a pre-exercise appraisal (which may include an exercise-tolerance test) and advice concerning the activities suitable for them. Most adults are cleared straight-away (by PAR-Q) to start an exercise program. As a consequence, PAR-Q cuts down on unnecessary visits to the physician by essentially healthy people and thereby can help slow the alarming growth in health-care costs.

Intensive medical and physiological evaluation of over 1,200 persons, and field tests on an additional 4,000 were used to ensure the accuracy of the questionnaire. Use by over 150,000 people with no untoward events substantiates the value of the PAR-Q approach.

PAR-Q is designed to be straightforward and simple, but it's an important first step, so don't rush through it.

- Read it carefully.
- Follow the instructions.
- Answer the questions.
- Follow the "yes" or "no" advice, whichever applies to you.

PHYSICAL ACTIVITY READINESS QUESTIONNAIRE (PAR-Q)*
A Self-administered Questionnaire for Adults

PAR-Q is designed to help you help yourself. Many health benefits are associated with regular exercise, and the completion of PAR-Q is a sensible first step to take if you are planning to increase the amount of physical activity in your life.

For most people physical activity should not pose any problem or hazard. PAR-Q has been designed to identify the small number of adults for whom physical activity might be inappropriate or those who should have medical advice concerning the type of activity most suitable for them.

Common sense is your best guide in answering these few questions. Please read them carefully and check the ☐ YES or NO opposite the question if it applies to you.

YES	NO	
☐	☐	1. Has your doctor ever said you have heart trouble?
☐	☐	2. Do you frequently have pains in your heart and chest?
☐	☐	3. Do you often feel faint or have spells of severe dizziness?
☐	☐	4. Has a doctor ever said your blood pressure was too high?
☐	☐	5. Has your doctor ever told you that you have a bone or joint problem such as arthritis that has been aggravated by exercise, or might be made worse with exercise?
☐	☐	6. Is there a good physical reason not mentioned here why you should not follow an activity program even if you wanted to?
☐	☐	7. Are you over age 65 and not accustomed to vigorous exercise?

*Developed by the British Columbia Ministry of Health. Conceptualized and critiqued by the Multidisciplinary Advisory Board of Exercise (MABE).
Translation, reproduction and use in its entirety is encouraged. Modifications by written permission only. Not to be used for commercial advertising in order to solicit business from the public.
Reference: PAR-Q Validation Report, British Columbia Ministry of Health, May, 1978.
*Produced by the British Columbia Ministry of Health and the Department of National Health & Welfare, Canada

YES
TO ONE OR MORE QUESTIONS

If you have not recently done so, consult with your personal physician by telephone or in person BEFORE increasing your physical activity and/or taking a fitness test. Tell him what questions you answered YES on PAR-Q, or show him your copy.

PROGRAMS

After medical evaluation, seek advice from your physician as to your suitability for:
- ☐ unrestricted physical activity, probably on a gradually increasing basis.
- ☐ restricted or supervised activity to meet your specific needs, at least on an initial basis. Check in your community for special programs or services.

NO
TO ALL QUESTIONS

If you answered PAR-Q accurately, you have reasonable assurance of your present suitability for:
- ☐ A GRADUATED EXERCISE PROGRAM—A gradual increase in proper exercise promotes good fitness development while minimizing or eliminating discomfort.
- ☐ AN EXERCISE TEST—Simple tests of fitness (such as the Canadian Home Fitness Test) or more complex types may be undertaken if you so desire.

POSTPONE

If you have a temporary minor illness, such as a common cold.

The PAR-Q advice to "postpone" if you have a temporary minor illness, such as a "common cold" deserves special mention. The rare sudden death during activity in otherwise healthy people is often due to viral infection of the heart muscle (known as myocarditis). Start your activity when you're healthy and ready for action and take rest breaks if you're ill and your body is asking for time off.

Undoubtedly, there will be a few who are unnecessarily advised to see their doctors, while some others may be cleared and then go on to experience some problems while exercising. For example, a positive response to Question 4 may have been the result of a short-term blood-pressure elevation many years ago, and even though things otherwise have been and remain quite normal, PAR-Q suggests consulting your doctor before starting. Follow the instructions. Give him a call. He may suggest you drop in for a quick check or merely say "Great idea, carry on." That's between you and your physician.

On the other side, there are those who get the green light but experience difficulty later on. Remember, PAR-Q clears you for "a graduated exercise program." This means starting comfortably and building up progressively—in short, "making haste slowly." It doesn't mean that the footballer of twenty years ago is ready for forty-yard dashes and stadium stairs. The former athlete must renew his interest just as the nonmover finds his new one—patiently, slowly, and intelligently. There's an important reason for this approach, and signs of overexertion suggest that further advice is imperative before continuing. Pains in the heart or chest, or spells of severe dizziness may indicate an inability of the heart to keep up with the demands of your activity. With the go-slow approach, the early part of the program, then, may uncover potential problems, about which advice should now be sought. Consider any of these warning signs as a "yes" response to PAR-Q and follow the appropriate advice. More details on warning signs follow shortly.

PAR-Q completed, you may be interested in one of the estimator fitness tests to find out where you stand. I don't suggest that everyone search out and try one of these tests before starting, because they aren't universally effective as motivators. Knowledge of your present fitness level, perhaps dramatically showing the need for improvement, may spur you to action. But testing is not the be all or the end all. It doesn't appear to weigh heavily in whether one is still active three weeks or three months hence.

One friend started and stopped his fitness routine several times, then signed up for another test "to get started again." I eventually talked him out of the test, we chatted awhile, and he decided he'd try some cycling. He knew he should start. Now he had to. He still needed motivation but, obviously, motivation of a different sort. I suggested he offer his kids a 15 per cent increase in allowance on one condition: They'd promise to take him on a bike ride each day when he returned from work.

Another friend shed an interesting light on the use of a retest (after some weeks or months of activity) for motivation and measuring improvement. He said, "I don't care if I've improved on the test; I feel better, and that's what's important."

If you're keen to see where you stand or to chart your improvement, there are some good tests. The 12-minute test, designed by Dr. Kenneth Cooper and popularized by his "Aerobics" program, is excellent. In his most recent book, *The Aerobics Way*, Dr. Cooper has added 3-mile walking, 12-minute swimming, and 12-minute cycling tests.

These tests can be quite strenuous, so it's important to learn how to pace yourself properly. Heed the name—12-minute walking/running test—and do just that. Run, but walk when you need to. Don't overestimate your abilities and start out too quickly.

Dr. Cooper cautions not to "go out and take the 12-minute test or other field test of fitness requiring maximal effort unless you are under thirty-five years of age, are already conditioned, or have progressed through at least the first six weeks of one of the programs." Consider one of the tests after you've spent adequate time reconditioning. You can then use that score as your bench mark to chart improvement.

The tests are easily self-administered. Walking or running tests are, perhaps, most accurately done on a quarter-mile track (most high schools have one). The idea is to cover the greatest distance you can in 12 minutes (or do 3 miles walking in as little time as possible). The walking, running, or cycling test must be done on level ground. Make sure you warm up and cool down with the test just as you would in a normal exercise session.

As previously mentioned in the discussion on PAR-Q, terminate the test if you have any warning signs of overexertion. Consult your physician before continuing with your exercise program.

The following charts outline fitness categories for various field-test results.

12-MINUTE WALKING/RUNNING TEST
Distance (Miles) Covered in 12 Minutes

FITNESS CATEGORY		AGE (YEARS)					
		13-19	20-29	30-39	40-49	50-59	60+
I. Very poor	(men)	< 1.30*	< 1.22	< 1.18	< 1.14	< 1.03	< .87
	(women)	< 1.0	< .96	< .94	< .88	< .84	< .78
II. Poor	(men)	1.30-1.37	1.22-1.31	1.18-1.30	1.14-1.24	1.03-1.16	.87-1.02
	(women)	1.00-1.18	.96-1.11	.95-1.05	.88- .98	.84- .93	.78- .86
III. Fair	(men)	1.38-1.56	1.32-1.49	1.31-1.45	1.25-1.39	1.17-1.30	1.03-1.20
	(women)	1.19-1.29	1.12-1.22	1.06-1.18	.99-1.11	.94-1.05	.87- .98
IV. Good	(men)	1.57-1.72	1.50-1.64	1.46-1.56	1.40-1.53	1.31-1.44	1.21-1.32
	(women)	1.30-1.43	1.23-1.34	1.19-1.29	1.12-1.24	1.06-1.18	.99-1.09
V. Excellent	(men)	1.73-1.86	1.65-1.76	1.57-1.69	1.54-1.65	1.45-1.58	1.33-1.55
	(women)	1.44-1.51	1.35-1.45	1.30-1.39	1.25-1.34	1.19-1.30	1.10-1.18
VI. Superior	(men)	> 1.87	> 1.77	> 1.70	> 1.66	> 1.59	> 1.56
	(women)	> 1.52	> 1.46	> 1.40	> 1.35	> 1.31	> 1.19

* < Means "less than"; > means "more than."

12-MINUTE CYCLING TEST
(3-Speed or less)
Distance (Miles) Cycled in 12 Minutes

FITNESS CATEGORY		AGE (Years)					
		13-19	20-29	30-39	40-49	50-59	60+
I. Very poor	(men)	<2.75*	<2.5	<2.25	<2.0	<1.75	<1.75
	(women)	<1.75	<1.5	<1.25	<1.0	<0.75	<0.75
II. Poor	(men)	2.75-3.74	2.5-3.49	2.25-3.24	2.0-2.99	1.75-2.49	1.75-2.24
	(women)	1.75-2.74	1.5-2.49	1.25-2.24	1.0-1.99	0.75-1.49	0.75-1.24
III. Fair	(men)	3.75-4.74	3.5-4.49	3.25-4.24	3.0-3.99	2.50-3.49	2.25-2.99
	(women)	2.75-3.74	2.5-3.49	2.25-3.24	2.0-2.99	1.50-2.49	1.25-1.99
IV. Good	(men)	4.75-5.74	4.5-5.49	4.25-5.24	4.0-4.99	3.50-4.49	3.0 -3.99
	(women)	3.75-4.74	3.5-4.49	3.25-4.24	3.0-3.99	2.50-3.49	2.0 -2.99
V. Excellent	(men)	>5.75	>5.5	>5.25	>5.0	>4.5	>4.0
	(women)	>4.75	>4.5	>4.25	>4.0	>3.5	>3.0

* < Means "less than"; > means "more than."

The Cycling test can be used as a test of fitness if you are utilizing the cycling program. Cycle as far as you can in 12 minutes in an area where traffic is not a problem. Try to cycle on a hard, flat surface, with the wind (less than 10 mph), and use a bike with no more than 3 gears. If the wind is blowing harder than 10 mph take the test another day. Measure the distance you cycle in 12 minutes by either the speedometer/odometer on the bike (which may not be too accurate) or by another means, such as a car odometer or an engineering wheel.

3-MILE WALKING TEST (NO RUNNING)
Time (Minutes)

FITNESS CATEGORY		13-19	20-29	30-39	40-49	50-59	60+
				AGE (YEARS)			
I. Very poor	(men)	>45:00*	>46:00	>49:00	>52:00	>55:00	>60:00
	(women)	>47:00	>48:00	>51:00	>54:00	>57:00	>63:00
II. Poor	(men)	41:01-45:00	42:01-46:00	44:31-49:00	47:01-52:00	50:01-55:00	54:01-60:00
	(women)	43:01-47:00	44:01-48:00	46:31-51:00	49:01-54:00	52:01-57:00	57:01-63:00
III. Fair	(men)	37:31-41:00	38:31-42:00	40:01-44:30	42:01-47:00	45:01-50:00	48:01-54:00
	(women)	39:31-43:00	40:31-44:00	42:01-46:30	44:01-49:00	47:01-52:00	51:01-57:00
IV. Good	(men)	33:00-37:30	34:00-38:30	35:00-40:00	36:30-42:00	39:00-45:00	41:00-48:00
	(women)	35:00-39:30	36:00-40:30	37:30-42:00	39:00-44:00	42:00-47:00	45:00-51:00
V. Excellent	(men)	<33:00	<34:00	<35:00	<36:30	<39:00	<41:00
	(women)	<35:00	<36:00	<37:30	<39:00	<42:00	<45:00

*< Means "less than"; > means "more than."

The Walking test, covering 3 miles in the fastest time possible *without running*, can be done on a track over any accurately measured distance. As with running, take the test after you have been training for at least six weeks, when you feel rested, and dress to be comfortable.

12-MINUTE SWIMMING TEST
Distance (Yards) Swum in 12 Minutes

FITNESS CATEGORY		AGE (YEARS)					
		13-19	20-29	30-39	40-49	50-59	60+
I. Very poor	(men)	<500*	<400	<350	<300	<250	<250
	(women)	<400	<300	<250	<200	<150	<150
II. Poor	(men)	500-599	400-499	350-449	300-399	250-349	250-299
	(women)	400-499	300-399	250-349	200-299	150-249	150-199
III. Fair	(men)	600-699	500-599	450-549	400-499	350-449	300-399
	(women)	500-599	400-499	350-449	300-399	250-349	200-299
IV. Good	(men)	700-799	600-699	550-649	500-599	450-549	400-499
	(women)	600-699	500-599	450-549	400-499	350-449	300-399
V. Excellent	(men)	>800	>700	>650	>600	>550	>500
	(women)	>700	>600	>550	>500	>450	>400

*< Means "less than"; > means "more than."

The Swimming test requires you to swim as far as you can in 12 minutes, using whatever stroke you prefer and resting as necessary, but trying for a maximum effort. The easiest way to take the test is in a pool with known dimensions, and it helps to have another person record the laps and time. Be sure to use a watch with a sweep second hand.

Another excellent self-administered fitness test, the Canadian Home Fitness Test, has been developed by Health and Welfare Canada. As the name implies, you can do it right on the stairs in your own home. It's a 3- or 6-minute step test (the less fit step only 3 minutes) done in time to the music of a long-playing record.

The field tests of fitness, previously mentioned, measure your fitness by how far or how fast you can go (which is why it's suggested you recondition before you try them). The Canadian Home Fitness Test, on the other hand, has you step at a prescribed pace. The test is age-adjusted, so the older you are the slower you step. This ensures that you don't overexert yourself, and it makes it a great test for those starting a fitness program. Your heart rate after the prescribed exercise indicates how hard you're working and, in turn, is used to estimate your fitness level.

The Home Fitness Test record comes in a package called the Fit Kit, which also includes a variety of other health and fitness material. Details at the end of the chapter indicate where the kit can be purchased.

Step Two
Planning

Now is the time for some thoughtful inaction. A fitness program requires an investment of time, which, at the moment, you may be able to think of better uses for. Purposeful planning means a better chance of your investment paying off. Consider the following four issues:

Time of Day

If you find beds extremely comfortable, if the choice of bed or exercise is no contest, don't fight it. You'll miss some nice sunrises, but there are other things.

There are a number of morning motivators. One finds he likes "to get it over with first thing." Another uses his morning run to plan his day at the office. A third wouldn't miss his morning outing for anything. It's nice to be out there when no one else is. Even big cities are peaceful if you pick the right time of day.

I once decided I'd run to work two mornings a week. This meant driving in the evening before delivering clothes, lunch, and my bicycle for the homeward trip. I lasted one day. The run was great. The trip the night before wasn't so good. A friend decided he'd ride to work, portaging suit, shirt, and tie; park his bike in the basement; shower, and proceed to the office. He was tougher than I. He lasted two days. Another cycler commutes five days a week. He rides only to and from work but covers ninety miles a week. He says he eats more now than he did in his prebike days when he was fifteen pounds heavier. The morning is for some, but not for others.

If window shopping leads to a budget overrun, then a noon-hour program could be your savior. If weight loss is on the mind, lunchtime activity burns off calories and takes your mind off eating. The midday workout also helps counter the two-o'clock drowsies.

The family man who finds it difficult to get away once home can use an after-work time to good advantage. Staying downtown for a workout can help you avoid the heavy, slow traffic. A one-hour workout may put you home just forty-five minutes later than usual. After one sortie into the morning world, the postwork predinner time remains mine. I find it a valued transition from the workday to an evening of leisure.

I envy those who find the nighttime theirs. Evenings are so fresh and clear and quiet. Some tell me their sessions leave them relaxed and ready for bed. I'd like to go then, but I feel so good after, there's no thought of sleep. Rumor has it that darkness brings forth the "closet jocks." Not wishing to reveal their new identity, they lurk about after dark.

There *is* a magic time of day to exercise, and it's *that* time that proves exactly right for you. Experiment and find a comfortable routine.

The Hassle Factor

Some activities are more accessible than others. You can walk, run, or cycle right from the front door. They require no travel time to and from participating. Swimming is usually not so easy. Make sure you want an activity enough that you'll put up with travel time if it's necessary. An extra half hour each outing may be just enough to make you decide it's not worth the effort.

Cycle commuting is a good trade-off and just right for some. The rationale is, if you must get there anyway, why not ride? Along with saving gas, wear and tear on the car, and parking money, you improve your health and fitness. If you live where bicycle paths abound, consider yourself fortunate. If not, gather your cohorts in fitness and lobby for bikeways and equal rights. If you start riding to work, you'll soon find that a shower at the office comes in handy. Unfortunately, these facilities remain frills in the corporate world. Get your boss interested in riding, and the frill may become a necessity.

Class Searching

There are two discernible groups—those who join a class and those who want no part of one. The joiner says, "I need a class or I just won't do it." The loner says, "Just tell me what to do and let me carry on."

If you're in search of a class, keep the following in mind:

- Choose one that suits your interests and aptitudes. Some programs label their classes by ability—"mild, moderate, and intense," for example. If you're entering a program like this, choose wisely and don't overestimate your abilities.

- Keep the hassle factor in mind. Travel time and business trips can make a class less appealing or totally inappropriate.

- Make sure it meets regularly. If it meets only once or twice a week, see if they give "homework." If not, plan some "homework" on your own.

- Make sure it includes warmup exercises and a cooldown, along with some endurance activity. (A recreational activity is a bonus.)

- Look for an instructor who is a teacher, not an entertainer. A valuable outcome of a class is that you and your activity are self-sufficient.

Some are loners by necessity, others by choice. The traveler, a loner by necessity, finds a one-man portable activity helpful. The loner by choice looks forward to his quiet-active time. Writing memos, answering the phone, or attending meetings are virtually impossible when you're out there alone.

Going it alone from the beginning can be difficult. For this reason, you might consider the semijoiner route. A neighbor or friend with the same aspirations is a lifesaver on days when you don't feel quite up to it. You can reciprocate and pull him along on his down days. The semijoiner group offers the best of both worlds. There's help when you need it, but if you miss today, you don't have to wait for the next class. Tomorrow is just fine. And you may enjoy the variety of alone and with-others days.

At some point in time, strive to be a loner. The camaraderie of the class makes it something special, but don't come to rely on it entirely. Don't always look outside for guidance and motivation. I've known many joiners who change jobs or cities and somehow don't find another class that fits in. Loners hardly miss a step during times of change.

Many loners come to cherish the silence and solitude their outings afford them. Joiners miss something very important if they don't sometimes go it alone.

Activity Choosing

What is sheer boredom and suffering for one is pure delight to another. The right activity offers at least some degree of enjoyment from the outset. Don't expect it to be instantaneously joyous, but neither should it be a dreaded bore. If you're absolutely and utterly convinced you're not a runner, then, for heaven's sake, don't go out and run to get fit.

The perfect match fits activity to your size, shape, and disposition. If quite overweight, you'd be wise to start with a weight-supported activity like cycling or swimming. If a torrid game of squash leaves you relaxed and refreshed, you've found your niche. If game's end finds you cursing yourself and your foe, you'd be wise to search around for something new.

A former military man reveled in the hard calisthenics issued by his instructor. Later he came to like a slow run and yoga. Keep an open mind. Experiment. Don't turn your back on the whole fitness world if one activity goes awry. There should be something for everyone.

Hard-core inactives heed this final word. If you've been through many years of little or no activity and now return searching for something quick, easy, and convenient, "Perhaps something I can do at home?," beware. Salesmen peddling exercise gadgets and equipment are waiting in ambush for you. More on this in Chapter Four.

Step Three
Precautions

Having contemplated the time of day, the hassle factor, class searching, and activity choosing, consider the following precautions:

Special Cases

Some people must take special care in program planning. For want of better terms, let them be called the "overweights" and "out of shapes," the "games" people, "old" people, and "problem" people. These terms are quite subjective and I don't particularly like them, but they serve to differentiate types of people and allow special advice to be passed their way.

First, the "problem" people. If you have any condition that could be aggravated or made worse by exercise, take extra caution. Remember, a "yes" response on your PAR-Q means this book is not to be your sole guide. Your doctor must help decide what's right for you.

If you have a known heart problem, for example, it's imperative that you seek medical advice before starting. The appropriate intensity and type of activity can then be prescribed. Many heart conditions respond positively to gradual and progressive physical activity. If your doctor's response is a hasty and emphatic "No activity," you may want to seek a second opinion. You'd be well advised to pick up a copy of the outstanding book *Heart Attack? Counter Attack!* by Dr. Terry Kavanaugh. Read it, then discuss it with a physician who thinks physical activity can play a part in the scheme of things.

Bone or joint problems may mean that some activities are more appropriate than others. Swimming and cycling, which support body weight, may be more expedient than running for starters.

Quite simply, medical concerns mean special precautions. It's an individual thing. Professional advice is your first move.

Next, the "overweights." You may be a few pounds above your preferred weight and have decided that this is the category for you. Or you may be considerably heavier than ideal weight but figure you're not so bad and "besides, one naturally gains a little extra weight as he gets older, doesn't he?" See how subjective it is.

At any rate, those who are excessively overweight (obese is the term used in health circles) should take special care in choosing their activity, just as those with bone or joint problems must. The extra weight means extra pounding on the joints. Perhaps you should walk now and save running for later when you've been active for a while and your weight has dropped closer to its ideal level. Or start with swimming or cycling, which support the body and are, consequently, more gentle.

We tread even more subjective ground when using terms like "out of shape" and "old" people. Out-of-shape stands in contrast to in-shape, and anyone starting a program is more "out" than "in." But fitness is not an either-or thing. It's a continuum with varying shades (or degrees) of fitness. You may call yourself "out of shape" but you're really just less fit than you'd like to be.

And what about the "old" people? Where stands this line between "old" and "young"? I know some "young" seventy-year-olds and many "old" people in their twenties.

If *you* think *you're* "old" or particularly "out of shape," take special note of the Intensity part of the FITTness Formula offered later in the chapter. It's to help you determine how hard to work and to ensure you don't overdo it.

Finally, advice for the "games" people. If you like fast action and competition, then pursue it. You have to do what's right for you. But make sure you're ready for the action.

Remember that athletes go to training camp each year to prepare for the coming season. If you're a former athlete making a comeback, you, too, must recondition and prepare for your endeavor. A period of exercises and some endurance activity could serve as your training camp. Racquet sports, for example, consist of fast stop-and-start movements requiring quick changes in direction. These put great demands on the ankles and knees. Make sure they're ready for it.

Take special note of the Type part of the FITTness Formula. Remember, also, that some activities are better than others. Your skill level largely determines an activity's effect on your fitness. If you're unskilled at tennis, play for fun but not for fitness.

Weight Loss

Three quick tips if you are looking for, or someone is trying to convince you of, shortcuts:

First, don't look for special exercises to lose weight in certain places. Spot reduction isn't possible. Certain exercises can increase muscle tone in specific areas but, unfortunately, they will not necessarily reduce fat in that area. Studies suggest that reduction is most likely to occur where fat deposits are most conspicuous regardless of the type of exercise pursued. The key, then, is expending more calories through activity than taken in food. If it's any solace, weight *usually* comes off first where it last went on.

Second, hard on the heels of the spot-reduction myth, comes the vibrators, massagers, and jiggly belts. Passive activity is a contradiction in terms. The case *for* vibrating, jiggling, or rubbing off excess weight lacks scientific evidence. You can't get something for nothing. (More accurately, you can't get less for nothing.)

Third, rubber suits to assist in weight loss are not only ineffective, they're also potentially dangerous. Temporary weight loss is possible. This is not a real loss but merely a water loss through increased, forced perspiration, which can result in dehydration. A rubber suit upsets the body's natural cooling mechanism, increasing body temperature, which can lead to heat stroke or heat exhaustion. Fluids must be consumed to bring the body back into balance. This returns body weight toward the pre-exercise level. Clothing should not be restricting but loose and comfortable, suiting both the activity and the weather.

Smoking

A *Financial Post* article "The Busy Slob's Guide to Semi-fitness," said, "It tends to be counterproductive to smoke just before, during, or after physical activity. Apart from that, if you can't say anything good about something, don't say anything at all."

Agreed. But further explanation seems prudent here. Along with increasing airway resistance, cigarette smoke increases the amount of carbon monoxide and carbon dioxide in the bloodstream, thus inhibiting the ability of the blood to deliver oxygen to the working muscles and putting a greater strain on the heart. At worst, smokers are wise to refrain for at least an hour prior to exercising. At best, they should stop entirely.

Drinking

Evidence suggests that there is a constriction of the coronary arteries with the consumption of alcohol. This is potentially dangerous prior to exercise since increased opening of the coronary arteries is essential to the oxygen demands of the heart. Abstention is wise for several hours before activity.

Pre-activity consumption of alcohol is additionally dangerous in cold weather as it tends to dilate peripheral arteries and increase the speed at which body heat is lost.

Pitfalls

Major pitfalls lie in overdoing it or "underdoing" it.

Dr. William D. Ross, in Chapter 18 of *Life and Health* suggests the following signs of overdoing it:

- A feeling of fatigue that does not leave within ten or fifteen minutes of finishing the activity.
- A feeling of tiredness that lingers after the workout. Drowsiness should not result. You should be relaxed, refreshed, and invigorated.
- Difficulty in sleeping.
- A buildup of fatigue. Workouts should not feel more difficult as time goes on. You should recover completely between sessions.

To these I add the following symptoms of "underdoing" it:

- Too many days between sessions. Don't procrastinate or make excuses.
- Giving in to mental fatigue. The desire for a snooze after a

day at the office usually comes from mental fatigue, not physical tiredness. Do not delay. Sitting and considering snooze vs. move is dangerous. Ninety-eight per cent of the time moving should win, and you'll be glad it did.

● A lull after a change. A change means that new routines and patterns must be developed. Fit your activity in from the very beginning. It'll be much harder later.

Warning Signs

The importance of listening to the body and heeding its warning signs cannot be stressed too strongly. Warning signs suggest that the activity is inappropriate or too demanding for your present fitness level.

The unfit should increase activity level gradually and slow down for uncomfortable signs—particularly *chest pain, undue shortness of breath, palpitations, and dizziness.* If any of these signs persist or recur, consider it a positive response on your PAR-Q and follow the "yes" advisory accordingly. Check with a physician before continuing.

Extreme soreness in joints and muscles also calls for reconsideration. Slight, transient soreness may occur initially, but should not persist. This "more than normal" soreness suggests the need for a reduction in the strenuousness of the activity. If signs remain, medical advice is warranted.

Warmup and Cooldown

An integral part of any exercise routine is a pre-activity warmup and a postactivity cooldown. The warmup consists of both preparative exercises and gentle activity. If you're a cyclist, for example, ride the first few minutes at slower-than-normal pace. Morning exercisers (especially runners) should take special care in warming up. You haven't had the day's activities to help you loosen up, so spend an extra few minutes stretching before you start.

Chapter Three deals at length with warmup exercises. For now, suffice it to say that slow stretching and strengthening exercises help raise heart rate, increase muscle temperature, stretch tight connective tissue at the ends of the muscles, and force lubricating fluid into the joints. The muscles can then work effectively through a wider range before discomfort appears. In short, the exercises and initial slow moving ready your body for the more demanding activities that follow.

Of equal importance is the postactivity cooldown. This is, again, a period of slow moving following your activity session. Five minutes is a minimum acceptable time for a cooldown. Runners should walk after the run, swimmers wade in the shallow end, and cyclists go the last part of the ride slowly (indoor cyclists continue pedaling with little or no resistance).

Standing still or sitting down immediately following your activity can result in blood "pooling" in the muscles most used during exercise. This deprives your heart and brain of much-needed blood and can result in dizziness or a light-headed feeling. Slow movement assists in efficient return of blood to the heart.

The cooldown should also include a return to some of the exercises done in the warmup. Concentrate on a few exercises that stretch the muscles most used during your activity session. For runners, this means Chapter Three exercises A-5, 6, 17, and 18, and B-5 and 17. Cyclists should return to A-5, 6, 15, and 16, and B-5 and 15. Whatever your activity you'll soon learn what muscles want stretching and, therefore, the most appropriate exercises to repeat.

Don't end your session with a burst or a sprint. It serves no useful purpose and, if overexerting, may prove dangerous to the very unfit. In summary, warm up leisurely, pursue your activity sensibly, then end slowly and peacefully as you began.

Step Four
The FITT*NESS Formula

F is for frequency or "How often?"
I is for intensity or "How hard?"

* The FITT acronym courtesy of Martin Collis, Ph.D., Physical Education Division, University of Victoria, Victoria, British Columbia.

T is for time or "How long?"
T is for type or "What activity?"

Frequency (How Often?)

Fitness cannot be stored; it must be replenished every couple of days. An old exercise adage suggests, "Three times a week is twice as good as twice a week."

Once a week may do more harm than good. The body never gets into the swing of things and may experience repeated postexercise stiffness, something that should only be an *initial* minor consideration. Injuries are more likely with a once-a-week routine. In addition, an exercise session followed by many days of inactivity allows the body to regress to its original condition before the next session comes around, thus never building up fitness.

A daily routine from the start may be equally unwise for many. There's no rush. The body will appreciate the reprieve an every-other-day routine provides. A daily session is not only hard on your body, it is also hard on your habits. You're trying to break into something new. Your program may be harder to sustain if you aim for a daily outing from the beginning.

An every-other-day or three-times-a-week routine is the wisest way to start. If weekends are a problem, try Monday-Wednesday-Friday. If the weekend is all right, go for an every-second-day program. Add more days later when you're ready.

Traveling can upset the training cycle, so plan road trips carefully. If you're a runner, look for a hotel near a park or other suitable running area. Don't dismay if hotel guests stare wide-eyed as you traverse the lobby in shorts and a T-shirt. They're likely with you in spirit. If you're a swimmer or indoor person, search out accommodations with a pool or exercise room.

Intensity (How Hard?)

Of our four-part formula, intensity takes by far the most abuse. Somewhere, a long time ago, a rumor started that if you don't finish your session huffing, puffing, red in the face, and looking for the nearest couch, then you didn't work hard enough. This rumor leads to trouble and, unfortunately, some still believe it. Any huffing, puffing, overfatigue signs mean overexertion—which can lead to stiffness, soreness, injury, and negative feelings about exercise. Instead of feeling refreshed and invigorated, you can end up tired. The whole purpose seems defeated.

Ex-athletes are the worst offenders. Brought up in a world of striving, dedication, and hard work, many find difficulty in coming to fitness with an open mind.

One holiday I traded jogging lessons for tennis instruction. The first day we ran, I said, "You run whatever pace you want and I'll tag along." I ran half as far as normal and ended up twice as tired. My partner finished with his usual sore legs. I said, "Tomorrow we run my pace." Next day we ran 50 per cent farther, it felt half as hard, and his legs didn't hurt. He was on to something new. (Incidentally, my tennis improved, mainly because he was an excellent teacher, but partly because I refused to let him tire me out on our morning runs.)

The impulsive types are almost as difficult to convert. They want results *now* and so they, too, aspire to the PTA (pain, torture, and agony) theory, dragged in from the athletic arena. This makes fitness a place where many visit temporarily and decide it's not a place they wish to stay.

The Make Haste Slowly movement is doing its best to pre-empt the PTA group. In this vein, one approach, popularized by Bill Bowerman, former University of Oregon track coach, is to exercise at conversation pace. Obviously not a method amenable to swimming, it has its place with hiking, cycling, running, and the like. He suggests that, for basic fitness, if you can't talk while moving, then you're going faster than necessary. Joe Henderson adopted for runners a term more common to another subculture. LSD, in running terminology, came to mean long, slow distance. Applicable to more than just running, it, too, suggests an intelligent approach to fitness training.

Inherent in conversation pace or LSD is "aerobic" activity. Aerobic in scientific terms means "with oxygen." In exercise circles, *aerobic* activities are those carried out at a comfortable, moderate level. Your oxygen supply meets the demands of your activity. This is to be differentiated from *anaerobic* (without oxygen) activities. Severe huffing, puffing, and straining serve to show you're exercising anaerobically. (You're not getting enough oxygen as you go along. Much recovery is necessary after stopping—like me on my hill.) It should be pointed out that many activities are potentially *aerobic* or *anaerobic*. It's really a matter of degree. A mild and moderate approach ensures aerobic activity; severe activity can be anaerobic.

There's a simple way to get you on the road to LSD, conversation pace, aerobic activity. Long used in the field of medicine, *pulse counting* gives some indication of stability of body function. (Pulse counting is what the nurse is doing when she holds your wrist and looks at her watch.) Adapted to the field of exercise, this monitoring of your heart rate gives immediate feedback on how your body is responding to activity. The nice thing about this technique is you can use it with any activity you choose.

There are two important tasks for now—learning how to count your pulse accurately, and understanding how hard to work in the beginning (that is, that pace that leads to good conversation). How to use pulse counting with specific activities is dealt with in later chapters.

Pulse Counting. The pulse is best felt with the index and middle fingers, not the thumb, as it has a pulse of its own and can throw your reading off. Gentle pressure is best. Pressing too hard can artificially slow the rate.

Two locations make counting an easy procedure. They're equally good, and practice will dictate which one is better for you. The first is the *radial artery,* which can be found on the palm side of the wrist in the hollow just below the base of the thumb. Bend one arm ninety degrees at the elbow, forearm extended in front, palm up, and the elbow resting against your side. Now locate the radial artery with the index and middle finger of the other hand.

The second place where the pulse is easily found is the *carotid artery* felt on either side of the neck about an inch back of the "Adam's apple." When taking the carotid pulse, there is sometimes a tendency to place the thumb on the neck on the other side of the "Adam's apple." This allows the possibility of a "squeezing" action on the throat. If you press with the thumb as well as with the index and middle fingers you can reduce blood flow to the brain which, in turn, can cause dizziness. To avoid this, don't cross over. Use the right hand for the right side of the neck, the left hand for the left side. In addition, too much pressure on the carotid artery can increase blood pressure and artifically slow the heart rate (giving an incorrect reading). The secret is gentle pressure with the index and middle fingers *only.*

The following diagrams show the locations of radial and carotid arteries and the proper technique for pulse counting.

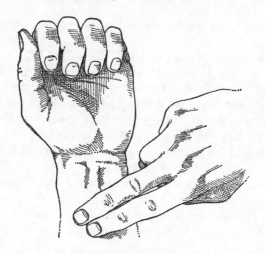

RADIAL PULSE

Starter Work Level. To begin, you should exercise at a level that elevates your heart rate to about 65 per cent or 70 per cent of your maximum. This level is high enough to reap endurance benefits but not so high that you'll approach the pain, torture, and agony threshold.

Some programs recommend working at 75 per cent from the beginning. This prescription often follows an exercise-tolerance test that determines *exactly* what *your* maximum capacity is. Since you'll be experimenting to find your capacity, better to err on the conservative side and start with 65 per cent or 70 per cent. If you find this too easy you can increase your work level accordingly.

What's a maximum heart rate? As a general rule of thumb, maximum heart rate is around 220 minus your age in years. Maximum pulse of the *average* 25-year-old is 195 (220 minus 25); that of the *average* 50-year-old is 170. This lower maximum rate results since the heart, like other muscles, loses some of its efficiency with age. Some of this natural loss is won back as fitness improves, so that a fit 45-year-old, for example, may have a maximum pulse rate some 10 to 15 beats above the 175 suggested for his age group.

The following "Fit Start" table suggests that the 25-year-old should exercise at 138 beats per minute to achieve 70 per cent of maximum; whereas the 45-year-old need only go to 120 beats per minute to reach this same 70 per cent.

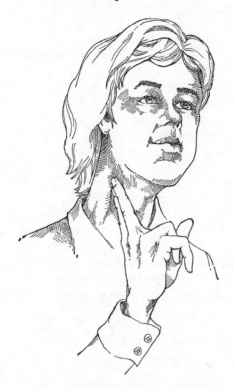

CAROTID PULSE

"FIT START" TARGET HEART RATES

Age*	25	30	35	40	45	50	55	60	65
Target Heart Rate In 10 Second Count	23	23	22	21	20	19	19	18	18
Equivalent One Minute Pulse Rate (=23 X 6)	138	138	132	126	120	114	114	108	108

*Use the nearest age group to your own. If you're under 25, use the 25 category. If you're over 65 extend the table, 70 year olds work to 17 beats/ 10 seconds, 80 year olds (you lucky guys!) work to 16, etc.
Target heart rates in this and the Keep Fit table are adapted from a paper *Heart Rate Monitoring: A Guide to Simplify Your Exercise Plan* by William D. Ross, Ph.D. and Raymond Duncan, M.D.

Note that pulse counting is done for *10 seconds*, a few seconds after stopping your exercise. There are two reasons for a 10-second count. First, it's long enough for accuracy. (A 5-second count, erring by a beat, means you're off by 12 in a minute.) Second, the count is meant to approximate your pulse rate *at the time of stopping*. Since your heart rate slows as you recover, a longer count isn't as accurate in approximating your rate right when you finished. The 10-second count offers a happy medium.

As you exercise it's not necessary to multiply your 10-second count by six each time in order to determine the number of beats per minute. If you're 30, you're aiming for a 10-second target rate of *around* 23; if you're 35, you're aiming for 22, and so on.

The target is not a magic number, etched in stone, only a general guide. If you're a couple of beats either side of the target and it feels good, that level is right for *you now*. If you're above average in fitness you may work quite comfortably a little above the target suggested for your age group. The overweight smoker may find a level below his suggested target more appropriate to begin. He can adjust upward later. Experiment and find the right pace for you. Remember, it should be a comfortable level. No huffing. No puffing. Just enough to start on the road to fitness.

Keep-fit Level. Later on, as fitness improves, you'll likely find you're working quite comfortably somewhere in the range suggested in the Keep Fit table. Don't rush to get there. Let it happen naturally. It can be a pain, torture, and agony level if you're not ready for it.

"KEEP FIT" TARGET HEART RATES

Age	25	30	35	40	45	50	55	60	65
Target Heart Rate In 10 Second Count	26	26	25	24	23	22	22	21	20
Equivalent One Minute Rate	156 (=26 X 6)	156	150	144	138	132	132	126	120

Again, the target is a guide, not a rule. A little above or below is just fine.

TWO FINAL CAUTIONS ON PULSE COUNTING. FIRST, DON'T BE CONCERNED WITH DAY-TO-DAY VARIATIONS.

BUSY TIMES AT WORK OR NOT ENOUGH SLEEP MAY TIRE YOU PHYSICALLY. YOUR ACTIVITY MAY FEEL HARDER AND YOUR PULSE RATE WILL BE CORRESPONDINGLY HIGHER. EXPECT—DON'T WORRY ABOUT—MINOR FLUCTUATIONS.

SECOND, PULSE COUNTING IS A VALUABLE TOOL IN THE EARLY STAGES OF A TRAINING PROGRAM, BUT DON'T OVERDO IT. AFTER A WHILE YOU'LL HAVE A NATURAL FEEL FOR THE APPROPRIATE LEVEL OF ACTIVITY AND WON'T NEED TO DO THE COUNTING ANYMORE. RELAX AND CARRY ON. AN OCCASIONAL COUNT FOR CURIOSITY'S SAKE MAY BE ALL THAT IS NECESSARY.

Some know intangibly how hard to work. They may not require the feedback that pulse counting provides. One nice thing about the pulse-counting scheme, though, if you're willing to believe it, is that it proves you don't need PTA to improve.

Now it's time for some practice:

- Line up a wrist watch with a sweep second hand. (The best watches are those that have sweep second hands that move in delicate 1-second intervals. However, any watch with a sweep second hand is adequate.)
- Practice finding both radial and carotid pulses while relaxing in a chair.
- After exercise your pulse will be faster than at rest. One of the beats will likely be right when you start to count. To make it accurate get in the habit of counting 0, 1, 2, 3 . . .
- Remember the *general* targets suggested for your age group, but be prepared to experiment and find your own personal target.

Time (*How Long?*)

Fifteen minutes' activity is considered a basic minimum to bring endurance-training benefits. Fifteen minutes' endurance activity, complemented by a 10-minute warmup and a 5-minute cooldown means a half-hour routine. Add to this a half hour for shower, clean up, and travel, and it's an hour per outing. Three sessions a week means 3 hours out of 168—or 1.8 per cent of the week. Hopefully, not too much to ask for.

Implied here is 15 minutes of *moving*, not necessarily 15 minutes of nonstop activity. For beginners, 15 minutes running or swimming may prove impossible. The secret, then, is to run or swim a little (aiming for your target heart rate), rest awhile, go again, and so on. Walking, hiking, and cycling may allow continuous activity from the outset. For now, just keep 15 minutes in mind. More details on time progression are offered in Chapters Four through Eight.

Some experts now suggest that 15 minutes is not enough. They say we should be looking at an hour daily of endurance activity. They're on to something, but, for the time being, I'll stick to the more traditional 15-minute theory. I'm comfortable with this approach for two main reasons. First, if an hour a day is issued as a blanket policy (add to this warmup, shower, etc., and you're at 1½ hours *daily*), then most of our potential recruits will say, "See you later, can't fit it in." By asking for too much, we may get nothing instead.

Second, as a teacher of fitness, I've seen how often one thing leads to the next. Many who start at 15 minutes soon find 30 more appropriate and desirable. In fact, as you progress you should slowly increase the duration of your activity, eventually closing in on a half hour. In time, a healthy percentage will be out there long enough to keep even the hour-a-day advocates happy. But to have asked for an hour from the beginning, some would never have started.

One step at a time. Start with fifteen minutes and see where it leads.

Type (What Activity?)

Activity choice has been discussed. Attention was paid to picking an activity that offers you some potential for enjoyment. If your approach is, "I don't like this activity but I know it's good for me so I'll try it," your routine stands little chance of lasting.

Further elaboration of activity choice is necessary. Since fitness is your goal, you must be selective in choosing. Some activities are more effective than others. The following activity hierarchy should help you keep things straight.

First comes the endurance activities. These allow you to work at a moderate level and sustain the effort over a period of time. They lend themselves to conversation pace and LSD. Included in this category are the universally available brisk walking, running, cycling, and swimming. Some people may have the good fortune of being able to canoe, hike, backpack, or climb. Winter means that others can turn to cross-country skiing, snowshoeing, and skating. In all these activities you can work up to your target heart rate and keep it there for the necessary length of time.

Next come a variety of recreational activities. These are characterized by fast action and stops and starts. Volleyball, basketball, hockey, badminton, and tennis have long been with us. Squash, racquetball, and handball have recently come into their own. A disadvantage of many of these activities is that skill level largely determines their effectiveness in improving fitness. Racquetball is fairly easy to pick up. It may provide good exercise the first time out. Squash seems to be an excellent conditioner. If your tennis is filled with many serves but few rallies, play tennis for fun but find something else for fitness. A further disadvantage of some recreational activities (basketball and hockey, for example) is that the game, not you, determines the level of activity. These fast, less controlled activities, if you're not ready for them, increase the chance of overexertion, injuries, and accidents.

If you're not sure what effect your sport's having, a quick pulse count can tell the story. Take a time out during the action. See how the count compares with your suggested target.

The third category includes golf, bowling, and other more passive recreational endeavors. They are fun, social activities that can have a practical effect on weight control, but they're ineffective for improving fitness.

What to Choose? If you're forty-five, have been inactive for some time, and favor squash, you'd be wise to consider a more gentle beginning. Let your body acclimatize slowly. Squash may prove a rude introduction. Warmup exercises and a progressive-endurance activity are more appropriate beginnings. Later, when a base of fitness has been built, add squash. It'll then be less tiring and more enjoyable.

If you're young, fit, and keen on recreational activities, you would still be wise to supplement them with something from the endurance group. Follow the old adage, "Get fit to play sports. Don't play sports to get fit." Remember, the suppleness and strength exercises of Chapter Three play their part in injury prevention, so if you really miss your game when deprived of it, exercises can help keep you playing.

Endurance activities are offered as the best starter activity for some, as an important supplement for others. They're also suggested for another reason. Recreational activities require a partner or a foe. Something may be lost with a companion. Games serve the physical. A solitary outing can be important for the spirit.

Just covered was much crucial information to help you start your program. In summary, think FITTness.

FREQUENCY	INTENSITY	TIME	TYPE
"Three times a week is twice as good as twice a week." Start with three or every other day. This ensures fitness maintenance. Personal preference may dictate more outings per week.	At the Fit Start or Keep Fit heart rate. Find *your* appropriate level of activity	Start with 15 minutes endurance activity and aim for 30. See how it goes. Experiment to find *your* optimum length of workout.	Strength and Suppleness Exercises for everyone. Endurance activities for all beginners. Later mix endurance and recreational activities if you so desire.

This ends Step Four. And while you're thinking FITTness and making final plans for starting, don't forget the final important item discussed in Step Three: Precautions—that is, a proper warmup and cooldown. The Chapter Three exercises form the basis of your warmup routine. Upcoming chapters outline exercises most appropriate as a part of the cooldown routine for each specific activity.

Step Five
Principles for Persisting

Starting is hard. Staying with it is considerably more difficult—evidenced by the large number of people who start but don't stay. The following principles are to help you to the point where there'll be no thought of leaving.

Patience

Persistence requires patience. As a rough rule of thumb on your road to fitness, look for about one month for every year of inactivity. Not to suggest a nonmover of twenty years will regain lost youth in a mere twenty months; this merely implies the longer you've been inactive, the more patient you must be. Age is no deterrent, but the older you are, the slower and more prudent should be your beginning. Recondition gradually; don't rush or force it. You're trying to turn this new activity into a habit that will stay with you for the rest of your life.

Expect changing motivators. You may start for physical reasons —because you know you should. It's as good a reason as any, but it won't carry you for long. Stay with it and you'll soon start to feel better for all your effort. You'll now be coming back for very practical reasons. With luck and *persistence* you'll get to the third stage where you're no longer in it for fitness. Oh, that comes anyway, but there's more to your activity now and you may find you can't go too many days without it.

Weight Loss or Not

A recurring theme since so many start for weighty reasons. Starting might be easy if weight loss is your goal. Motives are tangible and pressing. In the persisting phase you may find you're losing heart instead of weight.

The scale is not always your best guide. The mirror can help, too. Activity increases muscle tone. Muscle is denser than fat. That is, a pound of muscle is smaller than a pound of fat. You may be gaining muscle, losing fat, and losing inches. Your clothes may be loose, but the scales show you barely lighter. Don't dwell on the scale. Consult the mirror for moral support.

Remember that moderate exercise can mildly depress your appetite. Exercise in the few hours before eating can help you cut down at mealtime. But crucial to success is avoiding the 10 P.M. fridge raid to make up for what you missed at dinner.

If problems persist, consult a professional. Full weight loss advice is beyond the scope of this book. A nutritionist can tell you how to combine a dietary change and physical-activity program. Beware of "food experts" who are offering more than advice. Objectivity is often lost when you are being offered a bag of groceries along with food for thought.

Don't Rush

Set aside enough time for each session so there's no need to rush. Sufficient time includes that for travel, activity, shower, and return trip. Meetings and appointments pressing your session can make you a clock watcher. Extra time at the far end means you can run over a little if things are going well. I've ruined a few good runs because I left home to run somewhere specific, knowing I had to be there some minutes later.

Record Your Workouts

Buy a little book or use a month-per-page calendar. Get in the habit of writing down what you do. Once recorded, you'll remember exactly when you last worked out. Days unrecorded slip away more easily. Over a period of time, a record provides feedback on how you're progressing and gives a pleasant feeling of accomplishment.

Keep your book or calendar in a conspicuous place. This can help make you feel guilty for days missed. I don't really like the guilt idea as a motivator, but, at first, you may need all the help you can get.

A professor friend included a mood index and "ponderings" column in a training diary he prepared for his fitness classes. Joe Henderson's *Thoughts on the Run* grew out of postrun jottings in his training diary. This book was largely written while I ran. You, too, might want to record your own personal thoughts on the run.

Boredom

A math professor who once responded to my hitchhiking thumb said he liked to run on a track "simply because it's calibrated." I hope he's still running. The uncalibrated offers more leeway for change. A track can be confining. Seasons and the weather can do little to alter its sameness.

I have my favorite routes. The best takes in the oceanfront, a golf course, some shady residential streets, and its share of hills.

Another is less scenic but flatter. Some days, my legs appreciate the change. When these become too familiar, I go off exploring. But soon I return to my favorites. With the change, I appreciate them once again.

If a rut's your problem, change your routine. Head out at a different time of day. Change the mix of solitary to "with others" outings. Try another activity or do your regular program somewhere new.

Hollis Logue III, in "Eight Weeks to Start Shaping Up," said, quite simply, "Don't be a slave to Elm Street." Whatever your Elm Street, make some changes when it loses its fascination.

Injuries

The early part of your program will not be without its setbacks. While boredom may be easily rectified, injuries prove more troublesome. Injuries are an occupational hazard for the physically active. Athletes and fitness buffs are not unlike one another in this respect. Both must learn to heed signs of overexertion. The earliest indication of impending problems suggests a reduction in the amount of activity. See what the changes bring. If comfort returns, build up slowly and hope problems don't recur. Persistent problems mean that a change of routine or special advice is necessary.

Prevention is the wisest approach. Each person seems to have his optimum level of activity beyond which frustration waits. This optimum amount can be increased over time as long as you're slow and judicious in your approach. But there's no use planning for the Boston Marathon if your body is happiest with a dozen weekly miles at nine-minute pace. If an all-day bike ride lays you up, regular short rides to the store are more appropriate.

If prevention fails and injury occurs, intelligent, fast action can keep your recovery time to a minimum. The most common misfortunes are sprains, strains, and contusions. Sprains pertain to the joints, usually involving the ligaments. Muscles and tendons suffer strains. Contusions result from a blow, as in the common "charleyhorse." Inappropriate cycling could sprain ligaments in the knee; unprepared-for running can overstretch and strain a calf muscle; a collision on the squash court can result in a contusion of the thigh.

Keep the RICE formula in mind for treatment of injuries:

Rest

Ice

Compression (or pressure)

Elevation

Initial *rest* is important. A hasty return to action can put you back on the wounded list. Increase activity as pain and mobility permit.

Ice should be applied immediately, best accomplished by wetting the end of a tensor bandage, wrapping the injury with this part of the tensor, then holding the ice pack on with the remaining dry portion. The wet tensor acts as a conductor to draw in the cold. Plastic dry-ice packs are good. If you use ice cubes in a plastic bag, they should be replenished as they melt. Thirty to forty-five minutes is sufficient. After the initial icing, ice massage is the next step. Plastic styrofoam cups, filled with water and frozen, work well. The cup can be peeled away as the ice melts during massage.

Serious injuries, like strains in the calf or hamstring, should be iced every three or four hours during the day for the first forty-eight to seventy-two hours after injury. Less serious injuries should be treated with ice massage twice daily. Thereafter, alternating heat and cold treatment will help speed recovery.

Compression (pressure) applied with a tensor bandage helps contain swelling. Pressure should continue overnight and the next day. The wrap should be tight but comfortable. The day after injury, heat liniment can be applied to the area. It should be *rubbed on,* not *rubbed in.* No massage is recommended until the area is free from pain. (A cramp, on the other hand, *should* be handled by massage, loosening the muscle in question.)

Elevation plays its part, along with pressure, helping reduce blood flow to the area. Pillows under a sore leg usually end up on the floor by morning. A couple of blocks to raise the end of the bed are a better answer.

Minor injuries respond well to this treatment. Appropriate, immediate attention to problems hastens your return to action. More serious or persistent problems require longer recovery time and likely some sound medical advice.

If you're like me, not all doctors will do. There are still some who say, "Rest for a month and come back and see me if it still hurts." As an athlete in serious training, this advice falls on deaf ears. As someone who looks forward to his daily outing this advice is similarly frustrating. Some doctors understand athletes and other "movers." These are usually the ones who are active themselves and who have also developed an expertise in the area of sports medicine. Consult your local athletes to see who they go to. Take your troubles to him. Finding a sports-medicine physician you respect is important. Listening carefully and heeding his advice will speed your recovery.

This has been an important after-the-fact discussion—what to do when you're injured. The other side of the issue, injury prevention, is dealt with in upcoming chapters. Problems specific to various activities are considered in detail.

Rewards

Goals help some persist. Some programs offer rewards, like a T-shirt for regular participation, to help you get through the early part when it's not all ease and enjoyment. In a world where almost everything can be bought, there's intrigue in chasing something that can only be earned. Outside rewards help some get to the point where the activity itself is rewarding. Dr. Cooper's "Aerobics" program does just this. Earning your weekly points may be enough to keep you going in the early, trying part of a fitness routine.

If you respond to rewards and can't find a program offering any, set up your own. Convert weeks or months of persistence into something special you wouldn't normally do or buy. You're organizing the game, you decide on the prize.

Goals have their place, but they lead to an important crossroad. Goal achieved and still asking "What's next?" means some serious thinking is in order. If you're a few months into your program and you're still looking for external rewards to keep you going, you're in for trouble. People mismatched with their activity need enticements to make their relationship more palatable. Instead of asking, "What's next?" look around for a new activity.

The Right Activity

Already dealt with in detail, this issue is reconsidered because of its supreme importance. Step Two: Planning suggested you choose wisely. Don't start into something *only* because it's good for you. It must be appealing, too. Step Four: The FITTness Formula gave advice on proper activity choice for physical reasons. Some activities are better than others if fitness is a goal.

I worry when I hear, "I really *must* get back to the pool," and, "My husband says he's going to start skipping *again*." This starting *again* bothers me. Perhaps one should not "start again," but start anew. With luck and the right activity you need never start again.

A companionable activity is paramount. At first, companionship may be based on physical needs. The overweight may start out on a bike, the back-pain sufferer in the pool. But once basic fitness is achieved, few persist unless their activity remains important to them.

George Sheehan talks of one who ran with his neighbor every day for two years. The neighbor moved away and he never ran again.

I've known far too many indoor bicycle riders who exercised religiously for months, a holiday broke their routine, and they never rode again. I'm saddened by those who start and never make it. Almost all fail for the same reason. There was no joy and play in it.

Sociologists tell us play has meaning without purpose. We must learn to play. Far too many fitness routines are packed with purpose but devoid of meaning. You've made it through when your activity brings both meaning and purpose.

So now it's up to you. This chapter has brought you much crucial advice. Refer to the index at the front of the chapter to make sure you have everything clear in your mind before reading on. Chapters Four through Eight discuss various starter fitness activities. After considering the Chapter Three exercises, it's time to make a choice and get at it.

Finally, in all this talk, one nagging question remains: "How long?" How long must one persist? When does persistence, which implies working at it, turn to this ease, enjoyment, and joy that's spoken of? I wish I knew.

Where I went to camp, they read us a kind of riot act before we departed on canoe trips. Half in jest, it said, "If your canoe capsizes, hang on for three days and three nights. After that it doesn't matter."

On the road to fitness you must also hang on. It could be three weeks, three months, or more until you're no longer persisting, but just there. Numerous factors determine how long you'll wait for that day when it's "all as easy as a bird in flight." Age, years of inactivity, weight, smoking habits, and how faithful you are to your program play a part.

In the final analysis, rewards, training diaries, and partners to drag you along stand little chance of success stacked against an ill-chosen activity. To make it in the long haul there must be something in it that's right for you. When you find the right activity, enticements are unnecessary, obstacles prove no problem. Experiment. Play. It's yours to find. You'll know when it's yours for keeps.

Special Tips for Teachers

Starting and persisting are what teachers help people do. Some tips for them are in order before moving on to talk of specific activities.

The Chapter Three exercises can serve you well when conducting a group warmup before any kind of endurance or recreational activity. Remember that every group is made up of a number of individuals, and each participant is unique. Any beginner class, for example, will include a wide assortment of sizes, shapes, ages, and levels of "unfitness." Similarly, an intermediate class (however a program may define it) includes varying degrees of "intermediate" abilities.

If you say, "Do twenty situps," you're suggesting something that's largely inappropriate. Twenty situps will be just right for a few participants, too many for some, and not enough for others. Instead, say, "Let's do some situps." Each person can then do the number he wishes at the speed he desires. You'll soon learn how long to spend on each exercise—how long is enough and when straining begins.

This informal approach means each person works comfortably at his own rate. It has the added advantage of allowing you, as the teacher, to move around the class as they exercise, making individual corrections, offering advice, and giving encouragement.

This personalized approach is more difficult to achieve in an exercise-to-music class where teacher leads and participants move in time to the music. But there are still some ways to keep a session less formal and, therefore, individually appropriate.

When participants are sufficiently familiar with the exercises, you needn't always lead by example. You can start them on an exercise, then circulate as in the less formal approach, making corrections and giving encouragement. This makes it easier for you to see who is working too hard. Encourage them to take sufficient rest periods.

The in-time-to-the-music approach risks overexertion in some, while leaving others feeling the session was too easy. To counter this, you could have some participants work at double time, others at half time to the regular beat. The class will be less impressive to the spectator but more appropriate for all participants. If this proves too confusing, you must at least create an environment where participants feel comfortable about resting when they need it, when the pace of the class is a little ahead of them.

If the exercise-to-music class aims to improve stamina along with strength and suppleness, you should further individualize. Regular rest breaks and pulse monitoring can help each participant learn his or her own best work rate.

Ultimately, a teacher's greatest responsibility is ensuring that everyone feels good about how he's doing. Gently counsel the "make haste slowly" approach to those anxious to press ahead too quickly; support and encourage those who think they're falling behind. Create an environment where everyone feels comfortable working at his self-determined rate.

Consider the following suggestions for conducting group running programs:

Start in a gymnasium. It's warm and dry, so conditions are ideal. Inclement weather is a *real* obstacle to beginners.

Encourage coed, mixed-ability classes. Beginners can look ahead and strive to be like the veterans. Veterans can be both sensitive and helpful toward beginners, knowing they started once, too.

Use pulse counting to individualize. The less fit run smaller, slower circles in the gym; the more fit, larger and faster ones. Change directions regularly. Run in the opposite direction to the group sometimes. This allows you to more clearly watch individual responses to the exercise and caution those pushing ahead too quickly.

When you get out in a park or on a trail, start with an "out and back" routine. If the group is running 3 minutes, reverse direction at the 1½-minute mark. Those who were running faster and leading are now the "followers." At the end of 3 minutes they'll be back in a fairly tight group. This helps you for pulse monitoring or if you wish to talk and give instructions while they walk and rest.

Don't be a leader of the pack. That's like a lifeguard always in the pool, swimming ahead of those he should be watching. Run at the back with those who need and deserve encouragement and support. The ones up front need less help except, perhaps, the occasional "go easy" reminder.

Later, as they progress and are running for longer periods of time, small natural running groups will form. People of comparable abilities and levels of fitness can run together, covering suitable distances at fitting speeds. Encourage this but get them all together for the postrun cooldown. Group spirit is a great motivator for beginners.

If you wish to inject some noncompetitive competition, organize a predicted time run when the class is ready for it. We call ours tortoise races and dedicate them to tortoises everywhere. Each participant picks a distance and predicts how long it'll take him to run it. The winner is the one coming closest to the time he predicted beforehand. It's kind of a race, but speed is no advantage; pacing and luck are. In this race, slowest can be best. Some may wish real competitive running later. That's just fine. But let them decide if and when that's right for them.

This informal and individualized approach can and should be applied to any group endurance activity. Two lengths in the pool or two miles on the road cycling are not right for *all* members of a group at any given point in time. Use pulse monitoring to good advantage and let participants progress gradually and comfortably.

As a teacher of fitness, educate, don't entertain. The principles in this book can help you help others in a slow and sensible approach to fitness. But as you teach, program in *planned obsolescence*. With luck you'll become redundant as participants and their activities become self-sufficient. Your best measure of success is former class members coming back to tell you how well things are going, not a larger and larger group of people who *need* and want to stay with you.

Finally, remember that these adult-fitness principles apply equally to young adults. Schoolteachers can use a go-slow routine in any kind of fitness or active health program. More and more teachers are following this "first two minutes, then three minutes . . ." approach to running, for example, but some still say, "Oh, we have our kids run three miles a day." Asking most students to run three miles a day from the very beginning is like telling someone to play "Taps" the first time they ever pick up a trumpet.

On a similar note, a grading scheme that says fastest is best is equally damaging if physical education is meant to be education for life and if the program aims to nurture positive feelings about physical activity.

Cooper, Kenneth H., M.D. *The Aerobics Way.*
New York: Bantam, (1977), 312 pp.

The Fit Kit (includes the Canadian Home Fitness Test),
available from: P.O. Box 5100
                Thornhill, Ontario
                L3T 4S5
                $7.95

Kavanaugh, Terence, M.D. *Heart Attack? Counter Attack! A Practical Plan for a Healthy Heart.*
Toronto: Van Nostrand, Reinhold (1976), 231 pp.

CHAPTER THREE

The Stretch Bit

SUPPLENESS AND STRENGTH EXERCISES

WARMUP PRINCIPLES

Exercises Should Be Gentle, Slow, and Pain-free
Breathing Should Be Rhythmical, Exhaling on Effort
Do Bent-leg, No-help Situps
Practice the Pelvic Tilt
Be Wary of Some Exercises: Deep Squats,
Chest-constriction Exercises, Jumping Exercises,
Lateral Knee Stretching, Back Extension,
Specific Yoga Asanas
Be Cautious After Injury

WARMUP GUIDELINES

Format
Progression
Technique

SERIES A AND SERIES B EXERCISES

MUSCLES ARE the first line of defense against injury to the various joints of the body. Grocery bags, garbage pails, and lawn mowers subject the joints to a wide variety of stresses. Recreational activities further tax the joints, with the nature of the activity determining where the greatest stress is placed. Tennis and golf tax the shoulder and elbow, running exerts extra forces on the hip, knee, and ankle, and gardening and lifting focus stress on the lower back.

To assume their role as protectors, muscles must be sufficiently strong and supple. Strong muscles help stabilize joints and protect their attendant ligaments and tendons. Adequate suppleness allows the muscles to exert their forces through a wide range and to do their job well. The exercises that follow are offered as both a preparative and a preventive routine. They bring two of the three s's—suppleness and strength.

As *preparative* exercises they ready the body for action. Chapter Two pointed out how this works. Stretching and strengthening exercises increase heart rate and body temperature, stretch connective tissue at the ends of the muscles, and help lubricate the joints. The result is less stiffness from other activities. The American Medical Association's *Comments in Sports Medicine* states quite specifically, "For endurance exercise or sports participation, the onset of muscle soreness appears earlier without warmup and, thus, limits exercise capacity."

As *preventive* exercises, they aim to reduce the risk of injury. The emphasis is on exercises for the trunk region, since it is the foundation of all activity. If the muscles in this area are not sufficiently flexible or strong, ease and freedom of movement are limited. Turning, bending, and stooping are through a smaller range before signs of overstretch appear. Lifting is more onerous. Very often, weak stomach muscles in combination with inflexible muscles in the lower back are causes of problems.

Under normal circumstances, the stomach muscles work with the back muscles on both sides of the spine. They support the spine, acting much like guy wires holding up a tent pole. Weak stomach muscles mean two guy wires must do the work intended for three. Without the stomach muscles helping out, a forward tilt of the pelvis and curvature of the lower spine can result. This curvature puts an extra stretch on the muscles of the lower back, which is an added concern if they're already inflexible.

Strong stomach muscles are especially important in lifting and carrying. They allow the trunk to act as a firm column, more evenly distributing the weight and reducing the load on the spine itself. Weak stomach muscles increase demands on the back muscles and are often the root of low-back pain.

At first, the exercises might act in a corrective capacity, strengthening weak muscles and lengthening short ones. Later, they serve as a simple, efficient routine for suppleness and strength maintenance. They're best done before your endurance activity for the preparative reasons previously mentioned. But more than this, they're a quick, simple routine that can and should be done on a *daily* basis—first thing in the morning, while watching the news or whenever proves best for you. Chapters Four through Eight reiterate and highlight the exercises important to specific activities. Their preparative and preventive role are detailed at that time.

Warmup Principles

Exercises Should Be Gentle, Slow, and Pain-free

Slow, gentle exercises are the polar opposites of bouncing, jerking, or violent ones. A most difficult task is convincing people of the relevance of this pain-free, gentle approach. In the past, bouncing, jerking exercises were the order of the day. They followed the mythical principle, "If it hurts, it must be doing some good."

Studies have shown the fast, bouncing and slow, gentle stretching exercises both effectively improve suppleness. However, considerable evidence suggests that the bouncing approach causes muscle soreness and increases the risk of strained muscles in unconditioned people. The slow, gentle approach brings about quite the opposite result. As a warmup prior to other activities they help minimize stiffness and soreness and they reduce the risk of injury.

Suppleness exercises lend themselves to a stretch-and-hold, gentle continuous, or alternating side-to-side movement. The nature of the exercise dictates which approach is most appropriate. In any case the action is slow enough that the muscle being stretched relaxes and *gives* with the movement. A fast, bouncing, or jerking motion stimulates a safety mechanism known as the *stretch reflex*. In fast stretching movements, the muscle *knows* it may be overstretched, the stretch reflex reacts, and the muscle contracts to prevent over-stretching. This contraction slows the movement in an attempt to prevent injury. Muscle soreness results. Pain is the muscle's built-in indicator that overstretch is occurring. Slow stretching allows you to heed this warning and stretch no farther. With fast, bouncing exercises you may find out tomorrow that you overdid it today.

Stretch-and-hold or gentle, continuous movements prove best. Bouncing and jerking defeat the purpose and can cause problems.

Breathing Should Be Rhythmical, Exhaling on Effort

Breath holding and straining, most often accompanying strengthening exercises, are to be avoided. Breath holding during exertion increases the pressure within the chest cavity. This causes a rapid rise in blood pressure because of the extra force put on the arteries. This rise in blood pressure diminishes the output of the heart and slows the return of blood, via the veins, to the heart. This, in turn, leads to a rapid decrease in blood pressure.

This fast chain of events goes by the name of the Valsalva maneuver. Sometimes called the "snow-shoveling syndrome," it makes the news periodically when some unconditioned adult harboring undetected heart problems has a heart attack straining to clear away a heavy snowfall. Because of the potential dangers inherent in this action, those with high blood pressure and known heart problems should strictly avoid breath holding during exercises (as well as getting pre-activity advice from your physician, as previously mentioned).

All exercising adults should avoid the Valsalva maneuver because of potential nausea, dizziness, faintness, headache, and even short periods of blackout sometimes associated with it.

Strengthening exercises should be accompanied by controlled, rhythmical breathing, with an inhalation and exhalation on every repetition. Exhale on the effort phase, inhale on the preparation phase.

Do Bent-leg, No-help Situps

Re-educating people away from the bounce-jerk syndrome is difficult. An equally demanding task is that of teaching the proper situp technique. If you do situps now but you do them with your legs straight or your legs bent but anchored down (under the corner of your couch, for example), try a simple test.

Lie on your back, legs straight and hands at your sides. Do a couple of situps in this position. Next, do a couple with the legs bent, hands at your sides again, but have someone hold your feet down. Get a feel for how difficult this is. Now try them another way. Hands at your sides again, legs bent so your feet are flat on the floor but without someone holding them down. Feel more difficult? There's a reason for this.

When you do bent-leg, no-help situps (that is, without anchoring your feet), your stomach muscles are doing most of the work. Straight-leg or bent-leg anchored ones use the thighs and the muscles in the front of the hip for the first part of the situp. Since the purpose of the situp is to strengthen the stomach muscles, you compromise this goal doing straight-leg or bent-leg anchored ones. You get more for your time from the bent-leg, nonanchored variety.

Along with straight-leg situps, straight-leg lifts (lying on your back and lifting both legs off the floor at the same time) have long been used to improve stomach strength. There's a very important reason why both of these should be avoided. In both exercises, the stomach muscles contract to assist in stabilizing the pelvis, but it's the muscles in the hips that do most of the work. As these muscles contract they tend to hyperextend the lower back and further tilt the pelvis forward. These exercises, then, continue to strengthen the muscles in the hips, the stomach muscles remain *relatively* weak, and a curvature of the lower back (swayback or lordosis) may become even more pronounced. The irony is that low-back problems may begin or increase due to these exercises, which were originally thought to strengthen the muscles of the stomach.

The muscles that flex the hip remain strong from walking and stair climbing. To maintain proper posture we must achieve a balance of strength between these muscles in the hips and the stomach muscles. This balance is achieved through *proper* exercise. Bent-leg, nonanchored situps help. Other exercises offered in the following routine also play a part.

Now, you might say, "I can't do this method of situp without straining, and you told me not to strain. Where does that leave me?" A six-stage situp (Exercise A-10) is offered as part of the warmup routine. Experiment and find the right one for you *now*. It's the one you can do eight or ten times without breath holding and straining. Be patient and you'll move on to the more difficult stages as your stomach gets stronger.

Don't compromise for short-term success and tuck your feet under the couch. And don't listen to your friend who works out at the local gym. He may tell you he does his on an incline board with his feet held by a strap to stop him from slipping off. He's getting strong hip muscles. Your stomach muscles are getting stronger faster than his, and you're working on the correct balance of hip-stomach strength.

Practice the Pelvic Tilt

The pelvic tilt exercise (A-12) is a simple but important one that should be done daily. It's especially important if you have some degree of swayback (lordosis). It creates an awareness of the desired flat-back position as well as increasing flexibility of the lower back and improving strength of the gluteal (seat) and stomach muscles.

Start with the position shown in Exercise A-12. As your technique improves, progress so you're eventually doing the exercise in the straight-leg position. Later you can do the exercise in the standing position. The ultimate goal is to carry over this flat-back posture to standing and walking.

Be Wary of Some Exercises

Deep Squats. Any kind of squatting exercise—without weight for stretching or with weight for strengthening—that takes the knees beyond a ninety-degree bend should be avoided. These activities put an excessive stress on the knee joint itself in addition to stretching the ligaments that are meant to stabilize the joint. If squat exercises are done they should not go past the ninety-degree bend of the knee (that is, thighs parallel to the floor), and they should be executed with feet shoulder width apart.

Chest-constriction Exercises. Chest-constriction exercises such as pullups, pushups, and isometrics (strengthening exercises where the muscles contract but no movement occurs—for example, pushing palms together in front of the chest) should be pursued with caution. They are conducive to breath holding, straining, and the attendant dangers mentioned earlier. If you have high blood pressure or known heart problems you should avoid them entirely. All middle-aged adults who have been inactive for some time should avoid them in the early stages of their program. You might consider them later when a higher level of fitness has been achieved.

Jumping Exercises. Jumping jacks and other jumping exercises should only be done after the joints have been adequately prepared. They should be preceded by gentle suppling exercises that ready the body for this demanding kind of activity. Middle-aged beginner types would be wise to avoid these exercises in the early stages of reconditioning. They serve no important function and can increase the risk of injury.

Lateral Knee Stretching. Lateral knee stretching should be avoided. Exercises like A-16 and B-16 must be done with both feet pointing straight ahead and *flat* on the floor *at all times*. Shifting the weight to the inside border of the straight leg and/or pressing on the outside of the straight leg put undue pressure on the ligaments on the outside of the knee.

Back Extension. The back-extension exercise is done lying on your front, anchoring the heels, putting the hands behind the head, and arching the back. Done this way, without the arms supporting the weight of the upper body, its intent is to strengthen the muscles in the lower back. It's a demanding exercise requiring strong contraction of the back muscles and a vigorous backward bend. Inherent in this fast movement is the risk of overstretching and injury. Increased strength does result, but it can be accompanied by a shortening of the muscles. Shortened lower back muscles contribute to a forward tilt of the pelvis and poor posture, increasing one's susceptibility to low-back pain.

Some fitness programs use a back-extension exercise where the weight of the upper body is supported by the arms. With the palms under the shoulders the upper body can be raised *slowly* off the floor. This slower movement allows you to stop at the pain threshold, before overstretching occurs. With arm support, the exercise is a stretching, not a strengthening one. It thus avoids the inherent dangers of the more vigorous unsupported back arch. Even this gentle approach can exaggerate poor posture and the forward tilt of the pelvis that this series of exercises aims to correct. With a view to proper posture both types of back-extension exercises are wisely avoided.

Specific Yoga Asanas. Yoga was born in a culture and at a time where overweight and back problems were virtually nonexistent. Some yoga teachers have not adjusted to changing times and still include straight-leg lifts, severe back arches, and other exercises now deemed inappropriate for even the healthiest of backs. For example, the "snake," the "bent bow," the "wheel pose," and other similar exercises should be avoided. If you're interested in yoga, find a teacher who takes a conservative approach, someone who mixes modern scientific principles liberally with the traditions of yoga. In addition, remember yoga is *not* a *total-fitness* routine. It helps your suppleness and strength but does nothing for the most important fitness component—stamina. Look elsewhere for stamina activities.

Be Cautious After Injury

Exercises after injury can be helpful in recovery but should be approached with caution and, where possible, under the direction of a qualified therapist.

Strained muscles can be restrained easily if overworked in the early stages of healing. Gentle stretching exercises are best at first, followed by strengthening exercises as healing progresses. A ligament strain is a little different. Movement should be minimized in the early part of recovery, with light stretching exercises to be added when the injured area is ready.

An important note: Disc injuries cannot be cured by exercise. But if exercises can be tolerated without aggravation, they can strengthen the muscles that determine posture and in this way help ease the condition.

A final word of caution: If you are presently under professional care for a known back problem, work only on those exercises you have been instructed to perform. Later, the more general routine may be appropriate.

Warmup Guidelines

Format

Two sets of eighteen exercises are offered. A nice round number like fifteen would be nice, but it would have meant omitting some important ones. There is some overlap—a few exercises are included in both Series A and Series B. Some exercises are perfect to achieve a certain end. Therefore, best has not been compromised for the sake of variety.

FORMAT FOR EXERCISE SERIES A AND B

EXERCISE NUMBER	TYPE OF EXERCISE*	BODY PART EXERCISED
1-4	suppleness	arms, shoulders and upper body
5-6		hamstrings (ie. back of upper leg) and lower back
7-8	strength	stomach, trunk and hips
9	suppleness and relaxation	shoulders, arms and stomach
10-11	strength	stomach, trunk and hips
12-13	suppleness	low back and hips
14-18		legs

*Some exercises strengthen one muscle group and stretch another simultaneously. In these cases, the exercise has been placed under the dominant action.

Progression

Series A and Series B are not radically different, but the second is slightly harder than the first. Series A could be performed your first four to six weeks, Series B for the same time period following Series

A. Thereafter, you might pick and choose from the two routines to keep things interesting. They're set up in a way to make this convenient but correct. Choose from Series A and B but go through in the same 1-to-18 order. This ensures that all major joints and muscles are being exercised. This order also ensures that relaxing stretching movements follow strengthening exercises where the muscles have been contracting. The above chart shows the types of exercises offered and the body parts exercised. For example, exercises 1 to 4 of both Series A and Series B are suppleness exercises for the arms, shoulders, and upper body. Exercises 5 and 6 are suppleness exercises for the hamstrings and lower back . . . and so on.

Technique

The suppleness exercises are either the stretch-and-hold or *gentle*-movement type. The description under each exercise sketch includes the appropriate instruction.

Stretch-and-hold exercises can be made more difficult as you progress by holding the stretched position for a longer period of time. Initially, you may do five or six repetitions of each exercise, holding each repetition for four or five seconds. Later on, you may actually do fewer repetitions of each but hold them longer (ten-to-fifteen-second holds, for example). With time you'll be holding more extreme positions as well. Since the connective tissue will be getting more pliable you'll be comfortable stretching through a wider range.

Gentle continuous or side-to-side exercises are made more difficult by increasing the number of repetitions. Remember, go smoothly and slowly as far as you can *without* pain. On the side-to-side exercises, *return* to the other side—don't bounce back to the other side. Similarly, the strengthening exercises are made more demanding by doing more repetitions. As you get stronger you'll be able to do more of each comfortably. Eight to ten repetitions might be just right to start. Build up slowly from there.

Don't rush through your warmup. If you're at the Fit Start level you should aim for a fifteen-minute warmup phase. This is about a minute per exercise, which gives you time to look at the sketch and read the description, perform the exercise, and rest briefly before moving on to the next one. At the Keep Fit level ten minutes may suffice. But don't make it any less. A hasty departure on your run or ride without sufficient warmup may bring an unwanted rest period when you overstretch an ill-prepared muscle.

Each exercise description includes the following information:

> *starting position*
> *action*
> *nature of exercises*—stretch-and-hold; gentle, continuous, or side-to-side movement for the suppleness exercises strength exercises *imply* repetitions
> *points to watch for*

To simplify the starting-position descriptions, note the following terms:

> *prone* means lying on the front.
> *supine* means lying on the back with the back of the head touching the floor.
> *standing* implies feet shoulder width apart. Variations on this position will be stated specifically.

One last word on technique: If you do an exercise incorrectly you may not get the benefit it's designed for and it may even cause problems. (As an example, see the description for Exercise A-16.) For this reason the exercise descriptions are detailed and they outline a step-by-step progression. If you were in a class you could get corrections as you go along. You're not, so the picture and description must be sufficient to ensure proper technique.

Plan on half an hour the first time you try each series. This will give you enough time to experiment and learn the correct technique. If you've worked on it and some exercise hurts or feels wrong, seek help. Show it to a professional. A simple change in arm or leg position could be all that is needed. If it remains uncomfortable, eliminate it from your routine for now and, perhaps, come back to it later.

Series A and Series B Exercises*

SERIES A	SERIES B
1. Arm Circles	1. Arm Circles
2. Side Stretch I	2. Side Stretch II
3. Trunk Twisting I	3. Trunk Twisting II
4. High-back Strength	4. Arm Crossovers
5. Sit-reach	5. Sit-reach and Low-back Stretch
6. Low-back Stretch	6. Leg Crossovers
7. Hip Twist I	7. Hip Twist II
8. Headups	8. Situps
9. Prone Stretch	9. Swimming
10. Six-stage Situps	10. Stretch and Tuck
11. Side Leg Raise	11. Swinger
12. Pelvic Tilt	12. Knee Crossovers
13. Cat Back	13. Groin Stretch
14. Hip Stretch I	14. Hip Stretch II
15. Thigh Stretch	15. Thigh Stretch
16. Split Stretch	16. Split Stretch
17. "Gastroc" Stretch	17. "Gastroc" and Soleus Stretch
18. Soleus Stretch	18. Ankle Rock

* Many of the exercises used here are adapted from Dr. William D. Ross's Exercise Management course at Simon Fraser University and Dr. Fred Kasch's Adult Fitness program at San Diego State University.

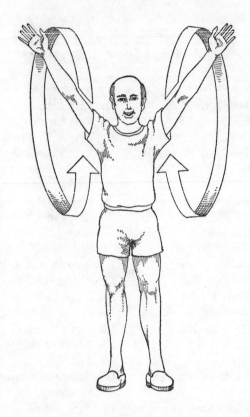

A-1
ARM CIRCLES

Starting Position: Standing, arms straight at sides, palms facing in.

Action: Full sweeping circles in a forward direction, reaching hands high above head and passing them close by the sides. Repeat the same movement in a backward direction.

Nature of Exercise: Gentle, continuous, circular motion.

Important Points: Keep arms straight, and do large, slow circles, not small, fast ones.

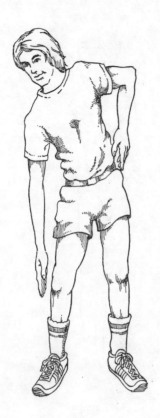

A-2
SIDE STRETCH I

Standing, arms straight at sides, palms facing in.

Reach the right arm down the outside of the right leg. Return to starting position. Repeat to left side. Alternate sides.

Stretch and hold.

Don't bend forward at the waist; instead, lean upper body to the side.

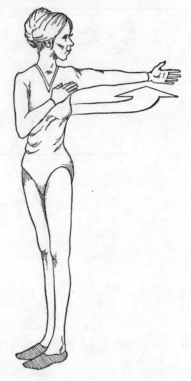

A-3
TRUNK TWISTING I

Standing, arms held straight at shoulder height.

Trunk twist to the right, sweeping straight right arm behind, bending left arm across your chest. Look back toward the right hand.

Repeat action to left side, left arm straight behind, right arm bent across chest. Alternate sides.

Gentle side-to-side movement.

Reach, *don't fling*, the arm back.

Keep feet flat on the floor throughout.

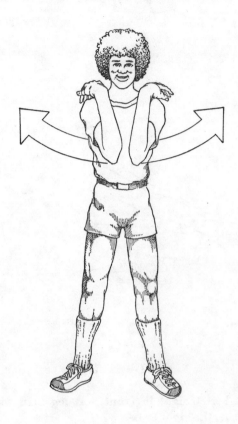

A-4
HIGH-BACK STRETCH

Standing, arms bent, fingertips resting on the shoulders.

Sweep arms in front, reaching elbows toward one another. Return to starting position. Sweep arms backward, reaching elbows behind.

Stretch and hold.

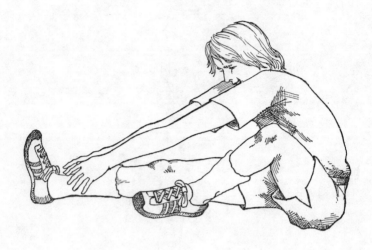

A-5
SIT-REACH

Seated, right leg straight in front, left leg bent with the left
sole resting near the right knee.

Reach toward the right foot with both hands. Hold. Sit up and
relax. Repeat a few times, then change leg positions and
repeat, stretching down the left leg.

Stretch and hold.

Reach *toward*, not necessarily *to* the foot—that is, don't overstretch. To take the pressure off the hamstring and lower back
between repetitions, place hands behind back and rest your
weight on the hands. When reaching forward do so with a
curled or bent, *not straight*, back.

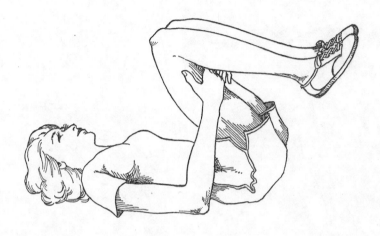

A-6
LOW-BACK STRETCH

Supine, legs straight and flat on the floor.

Bend the legs and pull the knees toward the chest, grasping the back of the thighs with the hands. Hold. Return legs to starting position and relax, then repeat.

Stretch and hold.

As the knees are brought to the chest, drag the heels along the floor to minimize pressure on the lower back. As the legs are straightened to the starting position, slide the heels on the floor.

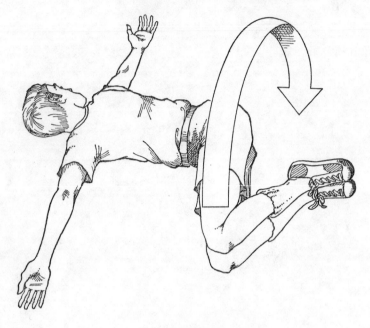

A-7
HIP TWIST I

Supine, legs bent, heels off the floor and near the seat, arms straight and flat on the floor at shoulder level.

With the knees together, roll the legs to the right, reaching the outside of the right knee toward the floor. Look toward the left hand. (This gives a better stretch and it helps you keep your balance.) Return to starting position. Repeat to the left side.

Repetitions. Gentle side-to-side movement.

The exercise can be made more difficult by holding the feet higher in the air. Don't go beyond a 90° bend at the hip *or* the knee, since this puts undue pressure on the lower back.

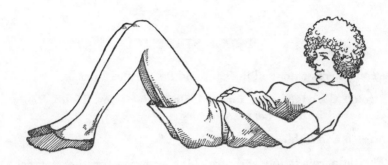

A-8
HEADUPS

Supine, palms resting on the stomach, legs bent with the feet flat on the floor.

Curl up, lifting the back of the head and shoulder blades off the floor. Look toward the knees. Hold. Return to starting position. Repeat.

Repetitions.

Hold only a few seconds. Exhale as you come up. No breath holding!

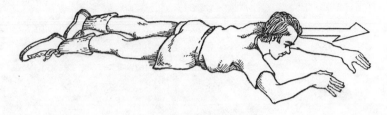

A-9
PRONE STRETCH

Prone, arms extended in front and flat on the floor.

Stretch the right arm forward along the floor. Hold. Relax. Repeat with the left arm. Alternate.

Stretch and hold.

This is a relaxation and stretching exercise for the stomach, arms, and shoulders. Keep the arms *flat* on the floor throughout (that is, stretch the arms forward *along* the floor, don't lift them up off the floor).

A-10
SIX-STAGE SITUPS

Supine, legs bent with feet flat on the floor.

Experiment to see which stage is appropriate for *you now*. They get progressively more difficult as you move from Stage I through Stage VI.

The stage that's right for you now is the one where you can do eight to ten repetitions WITH RELATIVE EASE AND NO BREATH HOLDING OR STRAINING. (YOU SHOULD EXHALE AS YOU COME UP.) DON'T BRACE AND SIT UP WITH A RIGID BACK. INSTEAD, CURL UP. (THIS PLACES LESS PRESSURE ON THE LOWER-BACK REGION.)

NOTE: If you must strain to do Stage I situp, then forgo situps for the time being. Start with A-7, A-8, and B-7, and add situps later when your stomach strength increases.

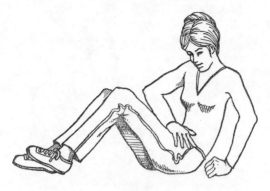

**A-10
STAGE I SITUP**

Curl up by leaning slightly to the right and pushing off with the right elbow. (This extra push helps you get started.) Roll back down, taking some of the weight on the right elbow again. Repeat, rolling up and back down on the left elbow. Alternate, pushing off with the right elbow, then the left. Exhale as you curl up, inhale on the way back down.

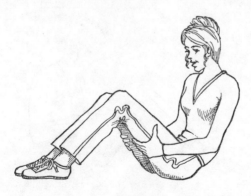

**A-10
STAGE II SITUP**

Curl up, grasping the backs of the upper legs. (This pull helps you get started.)

Curl back down. Hold the backs of the legs on the way down if necessary. Exhale as you curl up.

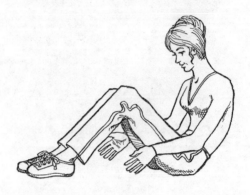

A-10
STAGE III SITUP

Curl up, with arms straight at the sides, but not touching the floor. Curl back down to starting position. Exhale as you curl up.

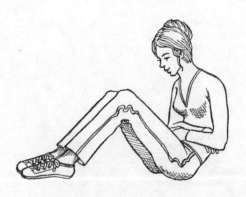

A-10
STAGE IV SITUP

Curl up, with arms crossed on the stomach. Exhale as you curl up.

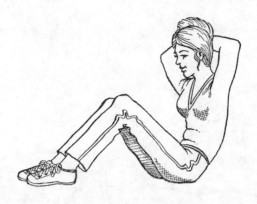

**A-10
STAGE V SITUP**

**Curl up, with arms bent and hands clasped behind your head.
Exhale as you curl up.**

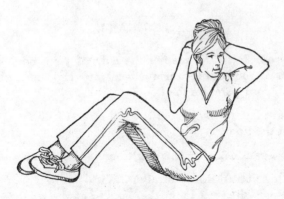

**A-10
STAGE VI SITUP**

**Curl up, with arms bent and hands clasped behind your head.
On one situp, twist the upper body so the left elbow reaches toward the right knee. On the next situp, twist so the right elbow
reaches toward the left knee. Exhale as you curl up.**

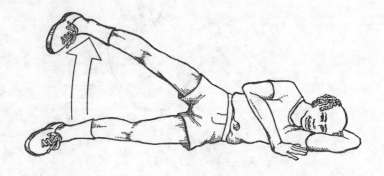

A-11
SIDE LEG RAISE

Lying on your left side, resting the side of your head on the upper part of the bent left arm. Place your right arm in front of you with your palm on the floor.

Lift the right leg up away from the left one with the toes pointing toward the floor.

Repetitions, gentle movement, don't bounce leg at the top.

Keep the leg you're lifting straight. With the toes pointed toward the floor, the muscle on the outside of the thigh is more effectively strengthened.

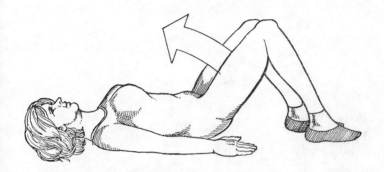

A-12
PELVIC TILT

Supine, legs bent, feet flat on the floor.

Press the lower back down flat on the floor, then rotate the pelvis by raising the buttocks off the floor.

Stretch and hold.

The lower back *must stay on the floor* as the buttocks are raised; otherwise, a bridge position is assumed and back extension may occur.

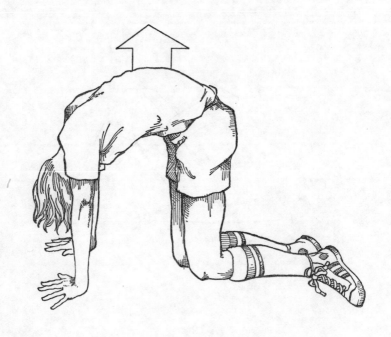

A-13
CAT BACK

On hands and knees, knees directly under the hips; arms straight and palms directly under the shoulders. Back flat (that is, parallel to the floor).

Arch the back, tucking the chin toward the chest. Hold. Return to starting (flat back) position. Repeat.

Stretch and hold.

Arms should stay straight, and arms and legs should not move (that is, no rocking forward or back). Return from arch to *flat back* position (that is, no sagging).

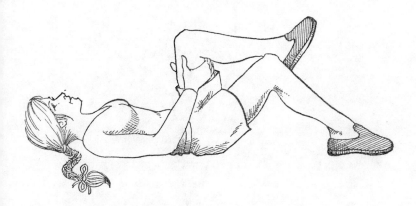

A-14
HIP STRETCH I

Supine, legs straight and flat on the floor.

Bend the right leg and pull the knee toward the chest, grasping the back of the thigh with the hands. Hold. Return leg to starting position. Repeat with left leg. Alternate legs.

Stretch and hold.

Press the lower back down flat on the floor as the knee comes toward the chest. Grasping the back of the thigh when the leg is held near the chest ensures that no undue pressure is placed on the knee joint.

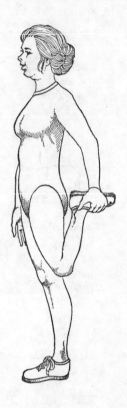

A-15
THIGH STRETCH

Standing, arms at sides.

Bend right leg, grasping the right foot behind, and pull the heel toward the seat. Hold. Return to starting position. Repeat with left leg. Alternate legs.

Stretch and hold.

Stand erect, don't arch the back as the heel is pulled in toward the seat.

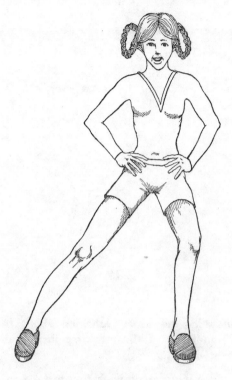

A-16
SPLIT STRETCH

Standing, legs more than shoulder width apart, hands on hips.

Keeping the upper body erect, shift the weight over the right leg (bending the right knee) while keeping the left leg straight. Hold. Return to starting position. Repeat to the left. Alternate sides.

Stretch and hold.

Keep both feet *flat* on the floor at *all* times. Shifting the weight to the inside border of the foot, when the leg is straight, places a great deal of pressure on the ligaments on the outside of the knee (and reduces the stretch on the muscles on the inside of the leg).

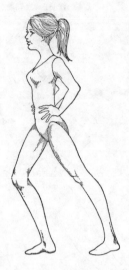

A-17
"GASTROC" STRETCH

Standing, hands on the hips, right leg about twelve inches (comfortably) in front of the left, feet flat on the floor and pointing straight ahead.

Keeping the upper body erect, rock forward over the right leg, bending the right knee, stretching the gastrocnemius (calf) of the straight left leg. Hold. Return to starting position. Repeat several times with legs in this position. Change leg positions (that is, left leg in front) and repeat to stretch right calf.

Stretch and hold.

Don't overstretch or hold too long in the early stages of your program. This is especially important if you regularly wear shoes with elevated heels, since these allow the calf muscle to shorten over time. It's important that the back foot points straight ahead and the heel stays flat on the floor throughout. Stretch only as far as you can comfortably, without the heel coming off the floor. Stretch by rocking the bent front leg forward, not by sliding the hips forward (which can put the lower back into an extension position).

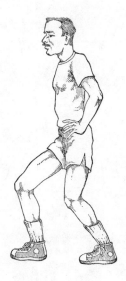

A-18
SOLEUS STRETCH

Standing, hands on hips, right foot about eight inches in front of the left, feet flat on the floor and pointing straight ahead.

Keeping the upper body erect, bend both legs, squatting slightly, thus stretching the muscle below the calf (soleus) of the left (back) leg. Hold. Return to starting position. Repeat several times. Change leg positions and repeat to stretch right leg.

Stretch and hold.

Don't overstretch or hold too long early in your routine. Ensure that the back foot is pointing straight ahead and the heel remains flat on the floor throughout.

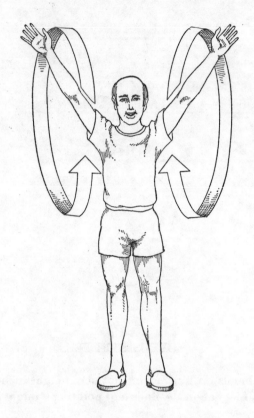

B-1
ARM CIRCLES

Starting position: Standing, arms straight at sides, palms facing in.

Action: Full, sweeping circles in a forward direction, reaching hands high above head and passing them close by the sides. Repeat same movement in a backward direction.

Nature of Exercise: Gentle, continuous, circular motion.

Important Points: Keep arms straight; large, slow circles, not small, fast ones.

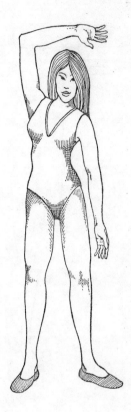

B-2
SIDE STRETCH II

Standing, arms straight at sides, palms facing in.

Reach right arm down the outside of the right leg, while reaching overhead and to the right with the other arm. Return to starting position. Repeat to left side, reaching right arm overhead. Alternate sides.

Stretch and hold.

Don't bend forward at the waist. Lean upper body to the side.

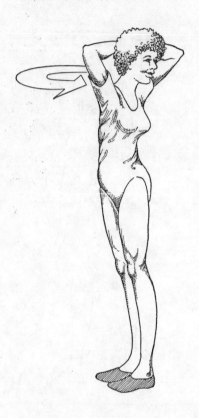

B-3
TRUNK TWISTING II

Standing, arms bent, hands clasped behind head.

Trunk twist to the right, looking as far behind as you can. Return to starting position. Repeat to left side. Alternate sides.

Stretch and hold.

Keep feet flat on the floor.

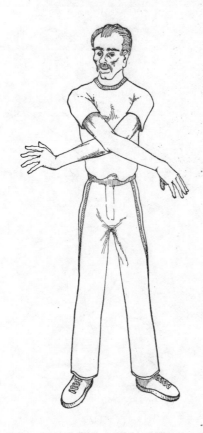

B-4
ARM CROSSOVERS

Standing, arms held straight near shoulder height.

Sweep arms forward, crossing them in front, then sweep them behind.

Gentle front-to-back movement.

Arms straight. Reach (*don't fling*) them front to back.

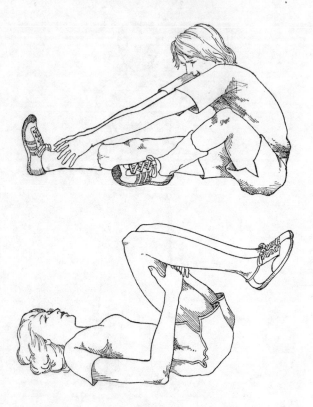

B-5
SIT-REACH AND LOW-BACK STRETCH

Seated, right leg straight in front, left knee bent with left sole resting near the right knee.

Reach toward the right foot with both hands. Hold. Then rock back pulling the knees toward the chest, grasping the back of the thighs with the hands. Hold. Return to sitting position with left leg straight in front. Hold. Alternate legs.

Stretch and hold in both positions.

As you go from the sitting to the back-lying position, drag the heel along the floor so the legs are bent when the feet leave the floor. (This ensures no undue pressure on the lower back.)

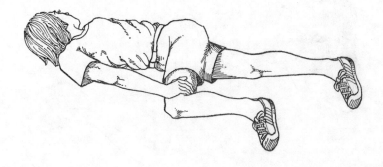

B-6
LEG CROSSOVERS

Supine, legs straight, arms straight and flat on the floor at shoulder level.

Bend the right leg so knee is up and right foot remains on the floor. Roll the right knee to the left so the inside of the knee reaches toward the floor. With the knee in that position, rest the left palm on the outside of the right knee and look toward the right hand. Hold that position. Return to the starting position. Repeat to the left side. Alternate sides.

Stretch and hold.

The knee of the bent leg goes toward, not necessarily to, the floor (that is, don't overstretch).

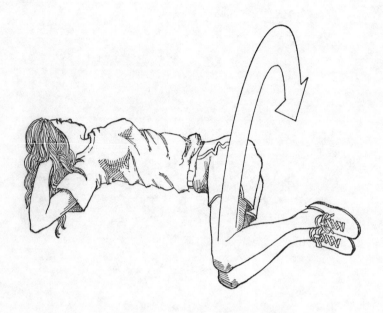

B-7
HIP TWIST II

Supine, legs bent, heels off the floor and near the seat, arms bent with hands clasped behind the head.

Knees together, roll the legs to the right, reaching the outside of the knee toward the floor. Look to the left. Return to the starting position. Repeat to the left side.

Repetitions. Gentle side-to-side movement.

No more than a 90° bend at the knee or the hip or you put undue pressure on the lower back.

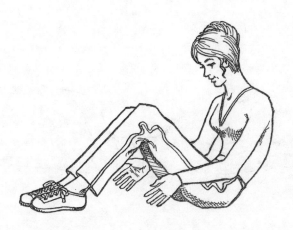

B-8
SITUPS

Supine, legs bent with feet flat on the floor, arms in position for the stage that is appropriate for *you now.*

Curl to upright position. Return to starting position. Remember, exhale as you curl up, inhale on the way back down.

Repetitions.

Don't strain. Curl up; don't sit up with a rigid back.

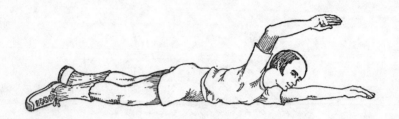

B-9
SWIMMING

Prone, arms extended in front and flat on the floor.

Roll your body slightly to the left, drawing the right arm down your side to the waist; then return it overhead to the starting position. Repeat, rolling to the right and pulling the left arm back and swinging it overhead (front-crawl motion).

Continuous movement alternating side to side.

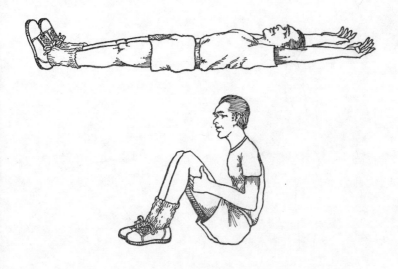

B-10
STRETCH AND TUCK

Supine, legs straight, arms flat on the floor and stretched out overhead.

Sit up and bend the legs simultaneously, arriving in a sitting tuck position with the hands clasping the back of the thighs. Reverse the action, returning to the starting position. Relax. Repeat.

Repetitions.

Drag your heels along the floor. This eliminates undue pressure on the lower back. Start the legs moving a little sooner than the upper body. This eliminates the possibility of starting into a straight-leg situp action. Curl the upper body up and down (that is, no rigid back).

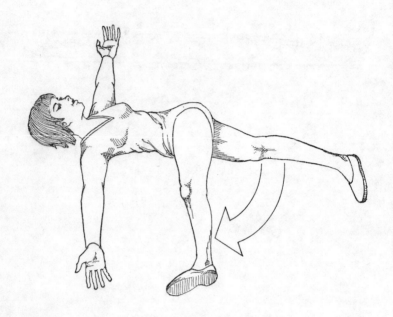

B-11
SWINGER

Supine, legs straight, arms straight and flat on the floor at shoulder level.

Lift the right leg slightly off the floor and, with it straight, swing it over toward the left hand. Return the right leg to the starting position. Repeat to the left side.

Repetitions. Gentle, alternating side-to-side movement.

Leg goes toward, not necessarily to, the opposite hand (that is, don't overstretch).

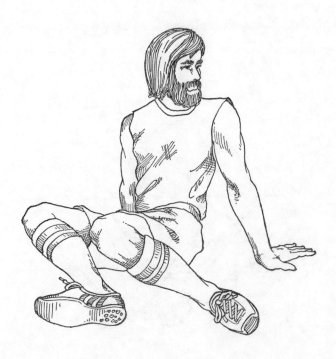

B-12
KNEE CROSSOVERS

Seated, legs bent, feet shoulder width apart and flat on the floor in front. Arms behind, straight, resting weight of the upper body on the palms.

Rock both knees to the right so the outside of the right knee and the inside of the left knee reach toward the floor. At the same time, look over the left shoulder. Hold. Return to the starting position. Repeat to the other side (that is, legs to the left, look to the right).

Stretch and hold. Alternate side to side.

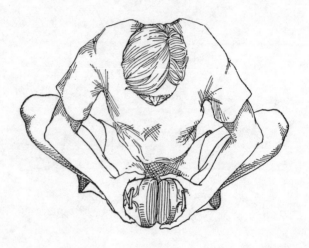

B-13
GROIN STRETCH

Seated, legs bent in front, soles of the feet touching one another, hands clasped around the toes.

Bend forward at the waist *with a rounded back* reaching the forehead toward the feet. Hold. Straighten up and relax. Repeat.

Stretch and hold.

The closer the heels to the crotch, the more difficult it is to bend forward. Find the position that gives a sufficient but comfortable stretch.

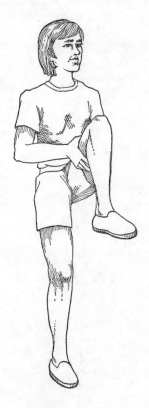

B-14
HIP STRETCH II

Standing, arms at sides.

Bend right leg at the knee and the hip, lifting the knee toward the chest, grasping the back of the thigh with your hands. Hold. Return to the starting position. Repeat with left leg. Alternate legs.

Stretch and hold.

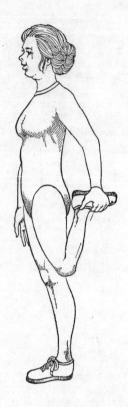

B-15
THIGH STRETCH

Standing, arms at sides.

Bend right leg, grasping the right foot behind, and pull the heel toward the seat. Hold. Return to the starting position. Repeat with the left leg. Alternate legs.

Stretch and hold.

Stand erect; don't arch the back as the heel is pulled in toward the seat.

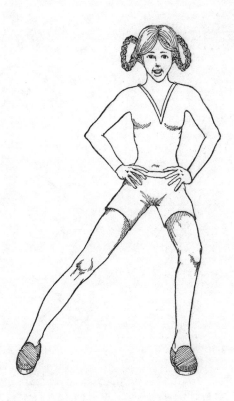

B-16
SPLIT STRETCH

Standing, legs more than shoulder width apart, hands on hips.

Keeping the upper body erect, shift the weight over the right leg (bending the right knee) while keeping the left leg straight. Hold. Return to the starting position. Repeat to the left. Alternate sides.

Stretch and hold.

Keep both feet *flat* on the floor at *all* times.

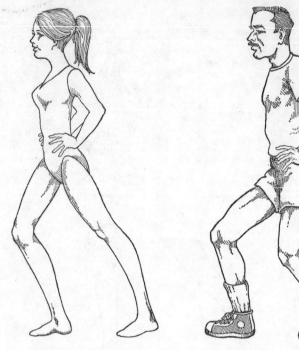

"GASTROC" STRETCH   **SOLEUS STRETCH**

B-17
"GASTROC" AND SOLEUS STRETCH

Standing, hands on hips, right leg about twelve inches in front of the left, feet flat on the floor and pointing straight ahead.

"Gastroc" Stretch: Rock forward over the right leg, bending the right knee, stretching the calf muscle of the straight left leg. Hold. Relax. Repeat. Do the same with the other leg.

Soleus Stretch: Move feet to eight inches apart, bend both legs, squatting slightly, stretching the muscle below the calf of the left (back) leg. Hold. Relax. Repeat. Do the same with the other leg.

Stretch and hold on both exercises.

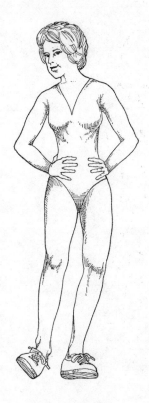

B-18
ANKLE ROCK

Standing, hands on the hips, feet together and flat on the floor.

Slowly rock the weight to one border of the feet, to the toes, other border, and heels. The knees should describe a circular motion. Do several circles to the right. Relax. Repeat in the other direction.

Continuous, gentle motion.

Don't lean forward at the waist—keep the upper body erect.

CHAPTER FOUR

Indoors

STATIONARY BIKES,
JUMP ROPE, AND
DANCING

INDOOR CYCLING
Bike Selection
Exercise Plan: Speed, Tension,
Distance, Progression
Further Suggestions: Saddle (Seat) Height,
Injuries, Cooldown, Thoughts on the Ride

JUMP ROPE
Some Tips: Equipment, Preparation,
Style, Progression

DANCING
Class Types
Class Searching

FIRST, a quick definition of exercise *gadgets* and exercise *equipment*. Gadgets are usually inexpensive items accompanied by claims of almost instantaneous fitness with little effort. All too many of these gadgets quickly go to their final resting place in the storage area. The salesman's richer and you're no more fit for your "little effort" and moderate expenditure. Don't waste your time or money on them.

Exercise equipment, on the other hand, does contribute to improved fitness if used properly. Equipment varies in cost, type, and complexity. Skipping ropes, rowing machines, and stationary bicycles play a part for those who enjoy this kind of program. Stationary bikes are discussed first, followed by some tips for "skippers." Rowing machines are not as common as stationary bikes, but the principles for an exercise program on each are the same. Consider the advice given for cycling to apply equally to rowing. (Remember the special-cases advice in Chapter Two. Rowing is primarily an upper-body activity, and so it may be inappropriate for some people.)

Indoor Cycling

The impressive annual sales of indoor bicycles shows that a significant number of people feel this is a logical place to start. If you think it may be the answer for you, consider the following advantages and disadvantages.

On the good side:

- It offers the ultimate in convenience—right *in* your own home.
- Conditions are ideal—rain, snow, and darkness are not en-

countered. It's a logical alternative for cyclists who face cold, snowbound winters.

● Hassles are minimized—traffic and stop signs don't exist; there's only your own dog to contend with.

● It's a quiet-active time where you can watch television, listen to the radio, or read.

On the bad side:

● Along with no rain, snow, or darkness, there are no birds, trees, or sunsets. There are no morning fogs or evening breezes. Every outing is totally predictable, virtually the same as yesterday and exactly what you can expect tomorrow.

If yours is a practical approach to exercise, indoor cycling stands a good chance of survival. But if you're the type for whom interest soon wanes, if a certain tedium that enters can outweigh the convenience, the ideal weather conditions, and no hassles, then indoor cycling may not be for you. Many indoor riders take up reading in self-defense. Reading makes the time go faster, they say. Some who ride indoors for physical and practical reasons soon find this not enough. Armed with magazine and music many never even make the hundred-mile mark on their "basement bike." The outdoor rider or the runner, on the other hand, finds reading both impossible and unthinkable. Reading intrudes on your thoughts and it comes between you and the sights, sounds, and smells unique to the day.

Decide on your approach to exercise and weigh the short- and long-term advantages and disadvantages. If indoor cycling seems right, then consider the following ideas on bike selection and program setup.

Bike Selection

Shop around and you'll come across "home" and "industrial" models. Industrial models are of rugged construction and cost about twice as much as home models. Industrial models are ideal for regular, heavy use in spas, YMCAs, and recreation centers.

Decent home models are not as abuseproof as industrial models but are quite adequate for home use. Get something that suits your pocketbook but make sure it has an odometer (mileage counter), speedometer, and tension adjuster. The tension adjuster is a dial, knob, or gearshift that allows you to alter the tension on the wheel and, hence, the effort necessary to push the pedals. A "calibrated" tension adjuster—standard on industrial models, not often on home models—indicates the *amount* of tension on the wheel. When you're shopping for a bike for home use don't worry about this feature. Home models are easily calibrated.

Finally, make sure that the bike is comfortable for *you* to sit on and that the saddle (seat) height is adjustable.

Exercise Plan

You'll have to experiment when you start. Your age, fitness level, and the type of bike you have will determine your appropriate combination of speed, tension, and work-rest intervals. The work-rest intervals go on the fifteen-minute moving theory (of Chapter Two). You'll pedal fifteen minutes, some working, some free wheeling with no tension (or resistance) on the wheel. Recovery sections, as shown on the Sample Workout Chart, are the rest intervals.

Using an outline like that on the Sample Workout Chart gives you a semiscientific approach. It helps standardize the work, ensuring that you follow the proper routine each time. In addition, it provides a place where you can note changes in your program as your fitness improves, and it serves as a tangible record of your progress. A five-by-eight-inch file card works well. Your workout chart can be on one side of the card, your daily record on the other.

Altering the *speed, tension,* or *distance* traveled, you can vary the difficulty of your program.

Speed. It matters not what speed you pedal as long as it's a natural rhythm for you. Some speedometers are in miles per hour, others in kilometers. If twenty miles an hour seems comfortable, start there. Later on, you may find yourself pedaling naturally at a faster rate. Riding the "mild" and "moderate" stages at one speed, the recovery, warmup, and cooldown a little slower, and the "speed" stage a little faster seem to work quite well. Don't settle on specific speeds too quickly. Experiment and find the best.

SAMPLE WORKOUT CHART

STAGE	SPEED	TENSION	DISTANCE	PULSE COUNTS
Warmup	15-20	1 turn	.5 mile	
Mild	20	2 turns	1.0	➤ 1
Recovery	15	No tension	.5	
Moderate	20	4 turns	1.3	➤ 2
Recovery	15	No tension	.5	
Speed	25	3 turns	.7	➤ 3
Cooldown	15-20	1 turn	.5	➤ 4 (2-3 Minutes after)

SAMPLE DAILY RECORD

ACTIVITIES	DATE 9/7	9/10	9/12	. . . .
Warmup Exercises	15 min.	15 min.	15 min.	. . . .
Cycling	15 min.	15 min.	15 min.	. . . .
Pulse Counts 1	18	17	18	
2	22	23	21	
3	24	25	24	
4	14	15	14	
Other Activities Skipping	2 min.	2 min.		. . . .
Cooldown	5 min.	5 min.	5 min.	. . . .

Tension. If you have a noncalibrated tension adjuster—a plain dial or knob that you turn—this is where you make your calculation. One turn of the knob may give you more tension than you'll ever need. If so, you might mark the knob in quarter- or eighth-turn segments. Other bikes might require two, four, or six *complete* turns to give noticeable differences in tension. It really doesn't matter how it works as long as you learn how much turning gives the necessary pedaling resistance.

How much tension to have on the wheel? How difficult should it be to pedal? This is where pulse counting comes into play. You should be aiming for the Fit Start or Keep Fit target heart rate (whichever is appropriate) as suggested in the charts in Chapter Two. You should be close to your target after the moderate or speed stage (pulse count 3 or 4, as shown on the Sample Workout Chart and Sample Daily Record). Raising your pulse too early (being at your target after the mild stage, for example) may result in fatigue. Warmup and cooldown should be with light tension, recovery periods with little or no tension, mild and moderate stages with mild and moderate tension (however your body defines them), as the names imply. The speed stage is done with a tension somewhere between the mild and moderate levels. Regular pulse counting in the early stages helps you find appropriate tensions. As fitness improves you can increase the tension during the mild, moderate, and speed stages accordingly.

Distance. Since your aim is to cycle fifteen minutes, not to cover any specified distance, the distance you travel in the early part of your program will be determined by your pedaling speed. If you're pedaling at twenty miles an hour, you'll go five miles in fifteen minutes.

It's merely a matter, then, of apportioning this total distance into the various stages. A half mile may be appropriate for the warmup and cooldown and two recovery periods, leaving three miles for the "work" phases. This could be divided: 1.0 mile "mild," 1.3 miles "moderate," and .7 mile "speed," as on the Sample Workout Chart. These are only examples for the various sections. The less fit might want longer recovery intervals, the more fit may reduce the recovery and sustain longer "work" sections. Later on you'll have both the desire and the ability for longer work intervals and shorter rest intervals.

Progression. Keep the FITTness Formula in mind. Three days a week is good to begin, but try to add more later. Intensity is increased by altering the pedaling speed, tension, and ratio of work to rest intervals. It's probably best to standardize speed and gradually increase tension and decrease rest (recovery) intervals. Time is the important factor. As in running, better to lengthen the session than keep it the same distance and make it more intense. Work toward a thirty-minute ride. Add a couple of minutes every two or three weeks.

Further Suggestions

Saddle (Seat) Height. Appropriate saddle height allows a slight bend in the knee when the ball of the foot is on the pedal, and the pedal is in the down position. A higher seat causes a side-to-side rolling over the seat as you reach for the pedal, resulting in an uncomfortable and inefficient ride. A seat too low, causing too great a knee bend, is equally inefficient. The thigh muscles, the power generators in cycling, tire too quickly.

Injuries. Injuries are less likely to occur here than in outdoor cycling. Cycling injuries are usually of the "overuse" type coming from many hours of riding. Long rides are unlikely on stationary bikes, so serious problems need not be expected. However, beginner injuries can result from insufficient warmup, so remember your exercises. They're as important here as anywhere.

Cooldown. The cooldown part of the ride should be followed by a few stretching exercises. A-6, A-15, A-16, and A-17 are excellent as a postcycling routine.

Thoughts on the Ride. Later on, if you're cycling more and enjoying it less, or cycling less and not enjoying it at all, prepare for a change. If the cycling itself is good but you're tired of your riding location, consider a transition to outdoor riding. Remember, boredom is self-inflicted.

Jump Rope

Jump rope (also known as skip rope or skipping) offers the same advantages as indoor cycling with one important bonus—it's highly portable. With your Chapter Three exercises and your jump rope you can go anywhere. It's a gymnasium in a suitcase and a logical answer for the businessman or anyone who travels regularly. Exercises and jump rope offer a maintenance program while on the road. As a lifetime activity it has the same shortcomings as indoor cycling. As a stay-in-one-place routine, adventures are few and monotony awaits.

Some Tips

Equipment. Fancy ropes with ball bearings in the handles make turning easier but more expensive. A wide variety of these ropes exists for the connoisseur. However, the old standard—No. 10 sash cord, available at your local hardware—is sufficient.

A proper length of rope should reach up under your arms when you stand on it. A little longer and you'll be able to maneuver better.

Preparation. Do your warmup exercises before skipping. Do an entire Series A or Series B but pay special attention to A-15, A-17, and A-18, and, if necessary, the telephone-book exercise (of Chapter Six) that strengthens the shin muscles. These are the working muscles when you skip. Skip in soft-soled, flat shoes on a soft surface (for example, a rug) if you can. Pay special attention to warming up the feet and ankles. (See Exercise B-18.) Return to these "special attention" exercises during your cooldown period.

Style. How to jump is up to you. The innovative mix things up with some fancy footwork. If you're short on ideas consult Peter Skolnik's *Jump Rope!* There you'll learn about the Heel-to-toe To-and-fro, Heel-to-toe Cross-as-you-go, and Back-to-back Thingumacrack. (You'll also learn the origin of "double dutch" and the lyrics for "Down in the Meadow" in North Carolina, Colorado, Delaware, Wisconsin, and Scotland.)

Unnecessary fatigue can result from two errors: turning too vigorously and jumping too high. Keep your arms close to your sides. Your hands should be no more than a foot from your sides. Turn with your wrists, not your whole arms. Jump only as high as you need to clear the rope. About an inch off the floor should do.

Jump on the balls of your feet and stay with a two-foot landing and takeoff at first. Let the knees bend slightly as you land. This gives a good cushioning effect.

Progression. As in any exercise routine, break in gradually. Start with two or three minutes' consecutive or "interval" skipping (that is, skip-rest) and add a minute or two each week. (A couple of minutes can be very strenuous. If you're quite unfit you might start with regular walking and add skipping later.)

Since you're just going a few minutes each time at the beginning, you could exercise five days a week instead of the traditional three. Skip three days, rest a day, skip two more, and rest another, and you're finished your first week! If you're huffing and puffing or your legs are getting tired, decrease the workload. Slow the rhythm or skip fewer minutes.

Some jump-rope books categorize speed levels by the number of turns you do per minute. Don't worry too much about fitting into a specific category. Experiment and find your rhythm. Seventy to eighty bounces per minute may be just right to start. Add more turns as fitness improves and when your legs, ankles, and feet are ready for them.

Dancing

New names abound as dance classes come into their own as viable fitness activities. "Jazz Fitness," "Rock and Blues," "Dancercise," and "Aerobic Dance" are relative newcomers beside the traditional ballet, tap dance, and others.

Many dance classes offer enjoyable, invigorating, and beneficial routines for improving fitness, but there are still a few that don't deliver what they advertise. Be selective in choosing the activity that's best for you. Shop around. Be wary of those groups that may offer "inches off in just weeks."

One fitness publication from England dealt with "slimnastics," (from slimming and gymnastics), offering it as "gymnastic and calisthenic activities done in a group." The name is appealing, especially for women, for it offers the prospects of both activity and weight loss, an enjoyable and worthwhile combination.

The book did offer some useful exercises but also included some erroneous advice, advice much desired by those seeking quick weight loss. On "spot reducing," it suggested wrapping a large, thin plastic bag around the offending area, to cause that area to perspire more profusely. It suggests, "This method has been used by dancers all over the world with great success." It even offers, "Banging the fat parts on the floor or a wall, and slapping them with the hand, breaks down the fatty tissue." One can only say, "Don't believe everything you read." To keep exercise and weight loss in the right perspective, consult the relevant sections of Chapters Two and Ten.

An educational seminar I once attended highlighted presentations by physiotherapists. They dealt with the "do's" and "don'ts" of exercise, focusing primarily on the "no-no" exercises like back extensions and straight leg lifts. They instructed why these shouldn't be done, what to do in their place, and emphasized the slow, gentle approach, as outlined in Chapter Three. One exasperated ballet teacher said, "You haven't left me any exercises I can still do!" It wasn't quite that bad, but the physiotherapist did show concern for some of the exercises she advocated.

Some ballet teachers, like their counterparts in yoga, are steeped in a certain tradition. Some still offer exercises now considered unwise even for healthy backs, and many still ascribe to the "bounce-jerk" approach to exercising. As mentioned in Chapter Three, studies suggest that fast, bouncing and slow, gentle stretching exercises both effectively improve suppleness. But the possibility of overstretching is greater with the bouncing variety, and with them comes an inherently greater risk of muscle soreness and muscle strains. This may present no problem for children or young dancers with strong and resilient muscles, but it is an obvious concern for inactive adults returning to fitness. A more gentle approach to exercises—like that outlined in Chapter Three—will prove a more sensible beginning.

Concerns covered, now consider class types and the following class-searching advice.

Class Types

Some types of dance are rightfully called endurance activities, while other, less demanding ones, are certainly fun but don't do much for fitness. Regional variations in names of classes, styles, and procedures make it impossible to say what's effective and what may need supplementing to ensure a total-fitness routine. However, some generalizations are possible.

A dance's place in the fitness hierarchy will depend partly on level of skill. In this respect, dance is like many recreational activities. Tennis is fun for the beginner, but fun *and fitness* for the intermediate. Beginning tap dancing may be easier than jazz fitness or aerobic dance, but as your skill improves and routines are learned, it could prove as demanding. Ballet has similar limitations to yoga. It's great for suppleness and strength, but in the early stages it does nothing for stamina.

If you're not sure of the endurance benefits of your routine, follow the advice given in Chapter Two to the "games" people. Take a break during your dance and do a quick pulse count. How does it compare to the recommended levels? If you're after total fitness, you now know if your dance is enough.

Class Searching

If you're looking for a dance class, keep the Chapter Two "class searching" advice in mind. In addition, consider the following:

Some dance classes include much hopping, bounding, and jumping. Look for a class that precedes these activities with a slow, gentle-stretching warmup. This slower warmup is important to prepare the joints and muscles for the demands of hopping and jumping.

Some dance or exercise-to-music classes use pulse counting throughout to ensure that each participant works at an individually appropriate rate. (A dance is followed by a walk [rest] interval and pulse count before the next dance is started.) This approach is especially important in classes where everyone exercises at the same rate in time to music. As mentioned in the Special Tips for Teachers section of Chapter Two, this "in time" approach can mean that the activity is too much for some, too little for others, and just right for the rest. A pulse count periodically during your session (in the early, reconditioning part of your program when you're still learning how much activity is enough) may confirm that you're overdoing it and remind you to go easy and take extra rest intervals. Or, if pulse counting isn't used, simply rest when you feel you need it. Don't do all the repetitions of every exercise if these prove too much for you.

Finally, select your class conservatively. Many programs advertise their classes as "mild, moderate . . ." and "beginner, intermediate . . . ," for example. Individuals approach a class with varying degrees of fitness or "unfitness," so any class will have a reasonable range of abilities. If you enroll in an intermediate class, for example, and no precaution (like pulse counting) is used to ensure individually appropriate activity, then the teacher will likely key the activity to the "average" fitness level of the group. You may or may not be "average," so the activity may or may not be entirely appropriate for you. Keep this in mind when you sign up. To avoid the possibility of overexertion, don't overestimate your level and enroll in a too-demanding class.

The three indoor activities here considered perhaps best exemplify the purpose-meaning discussion at the end of Chapter Two. Dance, at one end of the spectrum, can be totally playful and meaningful for those who participate. Riding a stationary bike, on the other hand, is totally purposeful but brings little meaning. Witness all those who start and soon stop and those who read, watch TV, or listen to the radio to reduce boredom.

So to the dancers, I say, "Dance on!" But remember: There are three s's to fitness, and stamina is the most important. If you don't get enough from your dancing, add another activity to your weekly agenda.

To the riders (and skippers) I say, "Beware." As short-term, on-the-road, or maintenance activities, they're great. But, in my experience, only 5 to 10 per cent of those who try are satisfied with stationary cycling or rope jumping as a long-term activity. If there's a chance you're in the other 90 to 95 per cent, before buying home equipment, try a walk in the park. Better yet, try a few walks. If walking isn't right for you, at least you didn't pay for the park. Be very convinced that home equipment is the answer before you pay up.

Skolnik, Peter. *Jump Rope!*.
New York: Workman Publishing Co. (1974), 157 pp.

CHAPTER FIVE

A Walking Start

WALKING AND HIKING

THE FIRST STEPS
Beginner City Walking: Progressing,
Style, Weight Loss,
Rewards

COUNTRY WALKING
Shoes and Boots: Boot Types,
Boot Fitting, Break-in, Care

Clothing: Socks, Pants, Tops,
Rainwear, Hand- and Headwear

Equipment and Supplies: Packs,
First-aid Kit, Map and Compass

Annoyances: Blisters, Sore Feet,
Sore Calves and Achilles Tendons,
Sore Knees and Thighs, Arch Pains

Walking Tips

BEYOND DAY HIKES

Two roads diverged in a wood, and I—
I took the one less traveled by,
And that has made all the difference.

—Robert Frost

WALKING IS a universal, easily accessible, nonprogram way to fitness. By its very nature, it begs the unscientific approach. There's no conscious thought of "exercising," but rosy cheeks, spring in the stride, and the good feeling after let you know you're on the right track.

The Sun Life booklet *Walking and Hiking* offers, "If you're looking for fitness, you'll be happy to know you can walk there." Walking doesn't offer the speed of running or cycling, or the demands of swimming, but it's equally pleasurable and relaxing, a great place to start, and, for many, a place they happily stay. And city walking can lead to country hiking, which brings with it a whole new set of rewards.

All you need are comfortable shoes and clothing to suit the weather and you can head out the door. View the advice offered here with a certain degree of detachment. Heed only what is useful to you now. Some of the guidance is aimed at longer walks and country hiking. It's given in the hope you'll head that way and, if you do, to help you set off properly.

The First Steps

Beginner City Walking

If you're a nonwalker now, start with two fifteen-minute sessions daily. At first, it may be difficult to snatch this time away from other "pressing" matters, so pick your times wisely and stick to them. You're trying to develop a habit, so don't let the alleged "pressing" matters encroach on this quiet-active time you've set aside.

Weekday walks for working people are easy to find. Get off the bus a few stops early or take a roundabout route between car and office. Use coffee time and lunch hour to good advantage. Walking, then, not only improves your fitness but also helps you avoid hazards such as extra calories and cigarettes.

Find a weekend routine that suits you. If you have a dog or dogs, condition them to regular walks. If walk time slips your mind, they'll remember for you.

Set a good pace. Strolling along isn't as good as walking briskly. Window shopping doesn't do it either. Your two fifteen-minute outings—at a suitable starting pace—should eventually grow to *the equivalent of* two half-hour brisk walks a day. One longer evening session may prove better for you. With luck and persistence this walking habit you're developing will become a daily looked-forward-to routine.

If you're curious about the distance you're walking, get a pedometer or do a trial walk to determine your pace. A pedometer, hung on your belt and adjusted to your stride length, will record your mileage (or "kilometreage," as the case may be). To determine your pace, time a measured mile or use a local quarter-mile high-school track. (Don't race, just walk your normal pace.) Thereafter, divide walking time by your normal pace to compute distance traveled. Later on, as your fitness improves, you may want to recheck your pace and adjust your calculations accordingly. Remember, *time* spent walking, *not distance* walked is more important, so do these calculations only if you wish—for interest's sake.

Progressing

Head for the hills when you're ready for them. Lean forward and shorten your stride on the upslope. "Braking" on the downhill can be tiring. Slow the pace and reduce stride accordingly.

Interval walking—alternating fast and slow segments—is another method to make the walk a little more demanding. You might even try Nathan Pritikin's "roving" approach outlined in *Live Longer Now*. Intersperse a few steps of running in your regular walks. One part running to a hundred parts walking may be just right to begin. If interest grows, change the recipe—sprinkle running less sparingly.

Style

Regular walking and hiking will lead you to a way of walking that's natural and best suited to you. Colin Fletcher says rhythm is the thing. That means a stride length and speed that are easy, unbroken, and comfortable. Walking's so automatic it frees your mind for other things.

Weight Loss

Walk on, safe in the knowledge that you and the joggers have a lot in common. Runners get a little more for their effort, but walkers and joggers expend about the same number of calories *per distance traveled*. A mile is a mile—walked or jogged.

Rewards

If you can do some utility walking—to shopping, to work, to school—think of your savings in bus fare or gas and parking. "Piggybank" your savings toward a future reward.

The best scheme I've ever heard of was devised by a lady who decided she'd walk daily (3½ miles each way) to the "Y" instead of taking the bus. She lost weight, got fit, saved her bus fare, donated to a "Y" scholarship fund, and was very, very happy. (Come to think of it, this may be the best approach to the reward scheme suggested in Chapter Two. You'll be rewarded enough already. Convert your success to someone else's worthy cause.)

Country Walking

Shoes and Boots

Leather shoes (offering good support) or running shoes serve city walking well. Leather shoes stand up better to wet weather. Running shoes are lighter, less tiring on long walks, and their thick rubber sole offers good cushioning on pavement. If you need running "walking" shoes, follow the shoe-selection advice for runners in Chapter Six.

For country walking, you'd be wise to move on from shoes to boots. (Some don't, though. I once met a girl who hiked in the Grand Canyon in the same kind of shoes I run in!) If you're buying your first pair, your best advice is "Don't overboot." Don't buy too much too soon.

Backpacking: One Step at a Time suggests four boot categories: "wafflestomper," trail, scrambling, and climbing boots. As you move from "wafflestomper" through climbing, the cost, weight, and complexity of the boots go up. Day hikers should restrict boot viewing to the "wafflestomper" and trail varieties.

Boot Types. Hiking boots reach up over the ankle. "Wafflestompers" are of light construction and have a reasonably flexible sole. They're billed as "good for casual walking" (that is, country walking and hiking).

Trail boots, intended for longer walks on tougher terrain, are heavier, and thicker and stiffer in the sole. Catalogues often describe them as "lightweight hiking" or "lightweight trail" boots.

The upper part of good boots are leather, either smooth, rough-out, or suede. Smooth leaves the leather the same way the cow wore it; rough-out boots are reversed, with flesh side out. Excellent boots come in both varieties. Quality of hide is more important than type of construction.

Suede is thinner, more porous, and "breathes" easier. It makes for light boots and is good for hot weather. However, its porosity makes it less desirable in wet weather. In all boots, the fewer seams the better—fewer places for water to seep in is much appreciated on wet days.

Soles come in a variety of designs, but virtually all good boots have a synthetic rubber-lugged base. Soles of lightweight boots are shallow, soft, and fairly flexible; heavier ones offer deeper soles with denser rubber.

Boot Fitting. Don't worry about the size. Be concerned only with how they feel. Different boots marked the same size may vary slightly. Snug, but not too snug, is what you're after.

They should fit "comfortably tightly" across the widest part of the foot, leaving about a finger's width of space in front of the toes. To measure the fingers width, stand up with the boot unlaced and slide your foot forward until your toes are touching the front. Slide your hand down behind the heel. One finger tight and the boots are small, two fingers in and they're loose. Somewhere between is just right.

With boots laced, the toes should be able to wriggle easily, but the heel shouldn't be able to lift up. Make sure you try on your boots with the same number and weight of socks you'll use for walking.

Break-in. You "break in" your body for longer walks. You must do the same with new boots. Wear them around the house. Go on short trial walks. The boots will be a little uncomfortable until you've worked out some of their stiffness and your feet begin to make an impression on them. Take care in this matter. Ill-prepared boots are major causes of blisters.

A "water treatment" is suggested for some of the stiffer boots. *The New Complete Walker* and *Backpacking: One Step at a Time* offer proper instructions.

Foam, rubber, or felt linings should be avoided. Some hikers like a leather insole, but anything more than this makes your boots less versatile. Built-in padding means less comfort in hot weather. Instead, add or subtract socks to get the desired amount of padding.

Care. Leather conditioning and waterproofing should follow purchase and precede use. Different boots require different kinds of treatment, so find out what yours need when you buy them.

Special care is necessary after muddy or wet hikes.

- Remove mud (it dries *on* and dries out the leather).
- Wash with a stiff brush and cool water.
- Spray the insides with disinfectant (this prevents mold).
- Stuff with crumpled newspaper or paper towel (this helps absorb moisture and helps the boot hold its shape).
- Leave to dry *anywhere but* near radiators, hot-air vents, etc. (excess heat encourages curling and dries out the leather).

Boots are like bodies. Properly treated and well-maintained they give reliable service. I have an eight-year-old pair of leather boots that are still trusty friends. I chuckle at the cost of my boots on today's market.

Clothing

Wool is hikers' material. It's resilient, absorbs sweat easily, and is comfortable and warm, wet or dry. It's the first choice from socks through tops.

Socks. Personal preference will dictate how many you'll wear. Opinions vary from one heavy pair to three light, with the consensus at two (one heavy, one light). Two pairs provide friction between the socks, reducing rubbing, thus minimizing risk of chafing and blistering.

An inner thin sock of cotton and an outer, heavier wool sock (reinforced with nylon) work well. The touch of nylon makes them more durable without detracting from wool's useful qualities. Some advice if you hole wool socks—have an "expert" darn them. Unevenness can lead to blisters.

Pants. Weather will determine the length, and preference and experience the kind of material. Loose-fitting pants allow free and easy action at the hips and the knees; tighter ones can restrict the stride.

Cotton is comfortable and warm when dry, but, once wet, offers no insulation or warmth. Cotton-nylon mixtures are light and strong, and more durable than cotton but offer less warmth.

Colin Fletcher reminds that pants should be tough since "chairs will be unpadded." His favorite material is corduroy (as long as it's good-quality) because it's warm, absorbent, and washes and wears well. And don't forget the value of wool on cold days.

Tops. A heavy sweater for warmth means you're stuck with an all-or-nothing approach. A number of thinner layers allows you to adapt gradually to changing weather, hiking speed, and terrain.

A cotton T-shirt is comfortable next to the skin. (Some use fishnet vests. Button up, and air is warmed and held close to the skin. Open up, and cooler air can circulate freely.) Wool shirts or sweaters—offering comfort and warmth—are good as second layers. Synthetic materials, because of their durability, are excellent for the outer layers.

Color of material is often overlooked but worth consideration. Colin Fletcher's advice, again, seems most appropriate. He suggests dark but bright colors, like orange or red. Dark doesn't show the dirt. Bright makes them harder to lose at a campsite or rest stop and makes you highly visible in hunting season or if you ever need to be rescued.

Rainwear. Rainwear selection necessitates compromise. If it's totally waterproof, it doesn't breathe, so you get wet from the inside out. If it breathes easily, it's barely water-repellent and lets the water in. Those living in the Pacific Northwest, facing incessant rain part of the year, lean toward the waterproof and are prepared to sweat a little. Your local climate might allow a water-repellent outfit—one that slows (not stops) the seepage of water in but doesn't make you as hot from the inside. Rainpants are handy for rest stops, bushwhacking or hiking through dense underbrush. Otherwise they make you hot. New rainwear, recently on the market and still relatively expensive, is advertised as waterproof but breathable.

Some hikers try for the best of both worlds with a poncho—a large rectangular sheet with a hole and a hood in the middle. Good ponchos have the hole slightly offset from the middle, so if you're carrying a pack the back of the poncho covers it. Air can circulate under, so you stay cooler. Some of the heavier models have drawstrings to reduce flapping in windy weather.

Plastic ponchos are inexpensive and completely waterproof. However, they don't "breathe" well and they tear easily. Woven synthetic fabrics like nylon are best. They're strong, light, and quite water-repellent.

Rainwear is a matter of personal choice. Some choose a poncho, while others say it's cumbersome, gets in the way, and they'd rather stay with a rainjacket. You must decide what's right for you.

Hand- and Headwear. With fingers in a common pouch, mittens prove warmer than gloves. Leather will do for moderately cold weather (however *you* define it), but you may want wool for colder times. (You can get leather with wool inserts.)

Hat style often reflects personality. Temperature and the presence of sun should also play a part in the material and style you choose. Hats are important in cold weather since much of the body heat is lost through the head. Sunglasses give added comfort on bright days and protect from snow glare.

Equipment and Supplies

Day walks into the country call for lunch, camera, and some extra clothing. You'll need something to carry them in.

Packs. The advice, again, is don't overdo it. *Walking and Hiking* says,

> Don't buy a super pocketed, multizippered monster pack if you're planning a few day trips carrying a couple of peanut-butter sandwiches.

However, it's better to buy a *slightly* larger pack and have it nearly full than to have an overly full small pack that rides hard on the back and bounces around.

Knapsacks or rucksacks come in cotton, cotton-canvas, and nylon. Nylon offers a good mixture of lightness, strength, and water repellency and seems the best bet. The better ones, with a bottom made of reinforced nylon, leather, or vinyl, can stand rough treatment. Cotton and cotton-canvas are heavier, can take more abuse, but are less water-repellent.

Look for a pack that offers a couple of small easy-access zippered pockets. They are handy for sunglasses, Band-Aids, and the like. The properly selected pack offers the advantage of multi-use, proving useful for cross-country skiing and cycling.

First-aid Kit. Carrying minor repair items is a wise precaution on day hikes away from civilization. Accidents can happen on a one-day outing just as they can on longer trips, so be prepared. Insect repellent and sunburn remedies should be included as well as supplies to deal with chafing and blisters.

Map and Compass. If you're going off the beaten track, a map and compass and the ability to use them can be lifesavers. Topographical maps are available from your local parks department or forest service; compasses are available at recreational equipment stores. Bjorn Kjellstrom's *Be Expert with Map and Compass* can teach you how to use them.

Annoyances

Runners and cyclists proceeding injudiciously encounter injuries. Walkers and hikers face what's more accurately called annoyances. Blisters and sore feet head the short list. Prevention is the key.

Blisters. Your first precaution is the proper boot break-in procedures discussed earlier. Second, heat brings blisters, so remove your boots, air your feet, and change socks whenever necessary. Pay attention to a "hot spot"—usually a sign of an impending blister. Downhill walking, with the feet sliding forward in your boots, can also be the cause. Tie laces a little tighter or add an extra pair of socks. In addition, soap flakes in your socks (or in your boots) and plastizote or other similar insoles in your boots help reduce the risk of blisters.

Remedial action for blisters requires tape, Band-Aids, or moleskin. (Moleskin is best, since it'll stick when your feet are wet.) If you feel a blister coming on, cover the area immediately (a "donut" helps protect the tender spot). Remove the covering at night to allow the air to get at it. Full blisters should be pierced on the downside of the bubble with a sterilized (for example, heated with a match) needle. Drain it completely and cover it. Keep it clean and change the dressing regularly to avoid the possibility of infection. If the loose skin puckers, remove it and cover the tender spot with gauze before putting on the moleskin covering.

Sore Feet. New boots may cause sore feet that don't develop to the blister stage. "House walking" and short walks help. Break them in well before venturing off on longer walks. Cut toenails short. Take regular breaks on longer day hikes—ten minutes every hour, a few minutes every half hour, or whatever routine proves best.

Hiking books don't include the following, but I add some measures to avoid two other possible annoyances.

Sore Calves and Achilles Tendons. Uphill walking, like uphill running, puts an extra stretch on the lower, back part of the leg. Hike fairly flat routes at first. Break into hill walking gradually. Stretching exercises A-17 and A-18 can help.

Boots are constructed with a heel slightly higher than the toe, but you may still need a heel lift. Heel wedges made of felt or foam inside the boot to raise the heel a little more also help here.

Sore Knees and Thighs. Downhill walking presents a different problem. Some books suggest running downhill. If you're new to hiking you'd be wise to start gently into this routine. The thigh muscles work hard as they contract to support the body weight on the downstep. Too much of this can leave your thighs fatigued and stiff. Fatigued muscles work less efficiently. They won't do their job, and more strain is placed on the knees.

Arch Pains. Pains in the arch are another potential hiking hazard. Some boots provide inadequate arch support. If you have problems, try inserting Dr. Scholl's Athletic A arch supports in your boots.

Walking Tips

Use caution when hiking in unfamiliar territory. Most hiking guidebooks recommend traveling with someone as well as leaving word of your whereabouts and expected time of return. Extra food, water and clothing, and a proper first-aid kit are helpful for unexpected delays or emergencies.

Consult local hiking booklets to learn more about new trails you intend to hike. Use them to get a *general* ideal of what to expect. They usually tell the length of trails and rank them with respect to difficulty. Be wary of guidebooks that tell you how long it takes to hike specific trails. Abilities and desired hiking speeds vary, so look only to trail-mileage guides and then approximate your own trip time.

Remember that a short, hilly hike can be significantly more demanding than a long, flat one. Let your hiking ability and your fitness level, not your desires, determine appropriate routes.

Take sensible precautions in very cold or very hot weather. Remember wool for the cold. Keep your head covered and button up tight at the neck during rest stops to keep in the heat generated during the walk. Make sure you have a dry change of clothes available. Use the buddy system to watch for hypothermia—the first signs being slurring of speech and clumsiness.

In hot weather, use sunglasses and a hat. Drink fluids regularly. If it's exceptionally hot, you'll need liquids every twenty to thirty minutes. Tomato juice is a good choice during and after activity. Also good are some commercial preparations, which include electrolytes (sodium, potassium, calcium, and magnesium) as well as vitamin C, all of which are lost in sweat. Be satisfied with a slower pace and don't go for longer than normal hikes on hotter than normal days.

One hiking book I read recommended asking permission before crossing private property. But Colin Fletcher says camouflage clothing in browns, greens, and grays is useful for such things as animal photography and *trespassing*. You choose!

I'll risk stating the obvious because it's so important. The country will only remain pleasing if we keep it that way. Leave only your tracks behind. Be careful with fires, and don't litter.

Beyond Day Hikes

Beyond day hikes is beyond the scope of this book. Colin Fletcher's *The New Complete Walker* and Harvey Manning's *Backpacking: One Step at a Time,* mentioned earlier, offer the advice and direction you'll need. Bjorn Kjellstrom's *Be Expert with Map and Compass* is a necessity if you wish to follow the roads "less traveled by."

Enough technical advice. It all leads to the more important point that walking gives a chance to look outward and, at the same time, turn inward. Walking's slow pace allows a full capture of the passing scene. I cherish the few days of snow each year that prohibit my bike ride to work. I head out early and, though I've gone this way hundreds of times before, my route seems, somehow, new. On the walk, you're in transit, neither here nor there, and so unencumbered.

Some walking places broaden the horizon of this outward look and add depth to the inward turning. I can't but turn to Colin Fletcher—master walker. He says it better than any. He talks of mountains, snow country, and other places. On the desert he says,

> You rediscover, every time you go back, the cleanness that exists in spite of the dust, the complexity that underlies the apparent openness, and the intricate web of life that stretches over the apparent barrenness; but above all you rediscover the echoing silence that you had thought you would never forget.

On the inward turning, he offers,

> Ten minutes' drive from my apartment there is a long grassy ridge from which you can look out over parkland and sprawling metropolis, over bay and ocean and distant mountains. I often walk along this ridge in order to think uncluttered thoughts or to feel with accuracy or to sweat away a hangover or to achieve some other worthy end, recognized or submerged. And I usually succeed—especially with the thinking. Up there, alone with the wind and the sky and the steep grassy slopes, I nearly always find after

a while that I am beginning to think more clearly. Yet "think" does not seem to be quite the right word. Sometimes, when it is a matter of making a choice, I do not believe I decide what to do so much as discover what I have decided. It is as if my mind, set free by space and solitude and oiled by the body's easy rhythm, swings open and releases thoughts it has already formulated. Sometimes, when I have been straining too hard to impose order on an urgent press of ideas, it seems only as if my mind has slowly relaxed; and then, all at once, there is room for the ideas to fall into place in a meaningful pattern.

Who could possibly add more?

Backpacker (bimonthly magazine)
65 Adams Street,
Bedford Hills, N.Y. 10507

Darvill, Fred T., Jr., M.D. *Mountaineering Medicine: A Wilderness Medical Guide.*
Skagit Mountain Rescue Unit, Inc. (1975), 48 pp.

Fletcher, Colin. *The New Complete Walker.*
New York: Alfred A. Knopf (1975), 470 pp.

Kjellstrom, Bjorn. *Be Expert with Map and Compass: The "Orienteering" Handbook.*
New York: Charles Scribner's Sons (1975), 136 pp.

Manning, Harvey. *Backpacking: One Step at a Time.*
New York: Vintage Books (1973), 356 pp.

ORGANIZATIONS

Alpine Club of Canada
P.O. Box 1027
Banff, Alta. T0L 0C0
Canada

The Sierra Club
1050 Mills Tower
270 Bush Street
San Francisco, Calif. 94104

CHAPTER SIX

Some I'll Remember

RUNNING

PREPARATION
General Warmup, The "Magic Six"

PROGRESSING
Pressing (Overdoing It) Now: The Semiscientific
Approach, The Less Formal Approach
Pressing Later

TECHNICAL TIPS
Surfaces
Style
Shoes: Selection, Care and Repair
Running Attire
Injuries: Shin Splints, Achilles Tendons
and Calves, Sore Arches and Feet,
Sore Knees, "Stitch"
Safety

There are no standards
and no possible victories except
the joy you are living while dancing your run.
In any life
joy is only known
in this moment—now!

> —Fred Rohé
> *The Zen of Running*

I USED the term jogger in Chapter Five, but I refuse to use it again. I have a strong aversion to this word. Jogger, to me, conjures up the image of some sort of second-class citizen, and there should be no class distinction in the world of running. I'll admit a personal dislike for the word, too. I'll never forget one day, as a high-school athlete, heading off from home on a training run and being accosted by my four-year-old next-door neighbor. She lounged on her front steps and yelled at me as I ran by, "Are you a jogger?" I had no answer for her. I ran off mumbling to myself.

One summer I had the good fortune of watching an all-comers track meet (you pay your quarter and run your race) in Eugene, Oregon. Several hundred participants completed the mile run for six-to-eight-minute milers. One middle-aged lady jumped for joy as she crossed the finish line breaking *her* magic seven-minute barrier. Are you going to call her a jogger? She's a runner if there ever was one.

Rumor has it that the speed at which you move determines whether you jog or run, and reports vary on the magic speed at which jogger turns to runner. I suggest, to keep things simple, that anyone going faster than a walk is running. Just because you like to go a little slower than the next guy doesn't make you any less a runner. The word jog, or its derivatives, will not be used here again. If someone asks, "What do you do to stay in shape?" answer with pride and assurance, "I run!"

If you're just beginning to run, expect to encounter good, bad, and indifferent days. If you've been inactive for a while or you're reasonably unfit, bad and indifferent days may dominate the early starting and persisting stages. This is only natural, it takes persistence to earn the special days.

Hollis Logue, in "Eight Weeks to Start Shaping Up," talks of this early stage:

> In a normal week, I enjoy two or three workouts from be-
> ginning to end. I have mixed feelings about another two or
> three. And at least one day each week, I ask myself, "Why
> did I ever start this stuff?"

The following guidelines aim to tip the balance, to help make the majority of your runs positive and to ensure you your share of special ones.

Preparation

General Warmup

Preparation means proper warmup. This, in turn, means emphasizing the exercises in Series A and Series B most important to running. The hamstrings, lower back, calves, and tendons must be sufficiently stretched before you go. In addition, the hips, groin, and muscles on the inside of the legs should be readied for action. Series A and Series B Nos. 5, 6, and 14 through 18 are "musts" before the run. I find it convenient to do these exercises along with the upper-body stretching exercises (Series A and Series B Nos. 1 to 4) before I run. Following the run, I do my strengthening exercises for the stomach and hips, but it also feels good to stretch the lower back and hamstrings again.

At the Fit Start level stay with the complete series in the proper order as a prerun activity. Later on, in the Keep Fit stage, you may find the exercise before and after routine more suitable. Beginner or advanced, you *should* do some gentle cooldown exercises. (A-5, 6, and 14 to 18 are excellent here.) As you increase your distance you will naturally feel the need for postrun hamstring and low-back stretching.

The "Magic Six"

George Sheehan has coined what he calls the "magic six" exercises for runners. If you run long distances (six miles a day, for example), you must heed the "magic six." Running strengthens the low-back, hamstring, and calf muscles. Without regular, proper stretching these muscles can become short and inflexible. Use exercises A-6 and 13, B-5, 6, and 13 to stretch the lower back; A-5 and B-5 for the hamstrings; and A-17 and 18 and B-17 for the lower legs. You should be doing an entire series (A or B), but do at least one of the exercises for each of these muscle groups and you've looked after the stretching half of the "magic six."

As running strengthens the muscles in the back and back of the legs, the muscles down the front—stomach, thighs, and shins—remain *relatively* weak. These muscles, in turn, must be exercised to ensure a proper balance of strength. Exercises 8 and 10 of both series help maintain stomach strength. A little cycling is an excellent way to maintain strength in the thigh (quadricep) muscles. In lieu of cycling, sit on a table with the legs hanging over the edge, bent at the knee. Hang a telephone book (except if you live in Los Angeles or New York!) or some similar object over your foot. Straighten the leg, return to the starting position, repeat a few times, then do the same with the other leg. This exercise strengthens the thighs to balance the running-strengthened hamstrings. To strengthen the muscles along the front of the shin (to balance the stronger calf muscle), start in the same table-sitting, telephone-book position. Instead of straightening the leg, merely flex the foot so the toes turn up toward the knee. Do a few repetitions with each leg. Alternatively, most recreation centers and Ys have a weight-training area. If you happen to run from there, you could visit the weight room briefly after your run a couple of days a week. Use their equipment for the two leg-strengthening exercises. Get a staff member to demonstrate the exercises and proper techniques.

That's the "magic six," three stretching and three strengthening exercises, which easily counter the strength-flexibility imbalance that can develop as running distance increases. The first four are for beginners and veterans alike. The last two strengthening exercises are important for distance runners.

Progressing

Pressing (Overdoing It) Now

The Zen of Running offers sound advice for beginners who want to press:

don't overdo it
underdo it
you aren't running because
you're in a hurry to get somewhere

Our noon-hour school-based fitness class sometimes finds us taunted by grade-three speedsters. In their own innocent way, they challenge us to press and overdo it. We plod along and they sprint ahead, tire, stop, and return to their seats in the bleachers. This always makes me think of some adults who start their programs in much the same way. They press on in search of instant results. Many tire, like the kids who race us, and fall by the wayside. There's no point trying to run a mile if a minute would be better. I encourage beginners to hold the tortoise in high esteem. Tortoises hang in there and usually make it.

How to progress without pressing? Consider the following: First, a semiscientific approach. The running times shown are not right for everyone. Some will progress more quickly. Others may wish to start more slowly. At any rate, the message is the same: "Make haste slowly." Be content to poke along, safe in the knowledge you're making inroads on fitness in a safe and enjoyable way. Why rush? What's a couple of weeks if you plan to be running for the rest of your life?

The Semiscientific Approach

Three times a week:

Week 1, Day 1—3 1-minute runs; 3 minutes running, 12 minutes walking=15 minutes moving. Heart-rate counting helps you adjust your speed to keep you near your target.

Week 1, Day 2—1-, 1½-, and 1-minute runs. Only 30 seconds more. Be patient.

Week 1, Day 3—1-, 1½-, 1½-, 1-minute runs; 5 minutes running, 10 walking for 15 minutes moving.

Week 2, Day 1—1-, 2-, 1½-, and 1-minute runs.

Week 2, Day 2—1½-, 2-, 1½-, and 1-minute runs.

Week 2, Day 3—2-, 2½-, and 2-minute runs equal 6½ minutes running. You should be starting to get a feel for *your* speed to achieve *your* target. And you're making progress.

Week 3, Day 1—2-, 3-, and 2½-minute runs. 7½ minutes running.

Week 3, Day 2—Walk/run ¾ mile. Get away from the playing field, explore new territory. Let your legs try out the pavement for a while.

and so on . . .

The point is: Don't press ahead every day; just move along naturally. Don't force your body; *allow it* to adapt to this new thing called running.

The Less Formal Approach. This is a similar but informal approach. Wind your wrist watch and head for the park. Note when you started. You're going to be moving for fifteen minutes. Run along, but walk when you feel you need it. Check your pulse. Above or below your target? Likely above if you wanted to stop for a breather. Walk and recover and run again when you feel ready. Think about the speed at which you were running. Try to run a little slower and come in closer to your target. If you do, it's likely you'll feel more comfortable and be able to run a little longer. Walk and rest again. Run again when you're ready. Fifteen minutes goes pretty fast.

Early in your program you may be walking much of your fifteen minutes. Later you'll be walking less and running more. Finally, you'll be running the whole fifteen minutes. At this point, don't turn your watch, which has been a helpful guide, into a scorekeeper. Some tend to stay at this same distance and try to run it faster and faster. Instead, reset your goal to twenty minutes running. You may have to slow the pace and walk a little to get there, but by now you've learned to be patient (?!). Later you may want to reset for thirty minutes. Remember: LSD, conversation pace is what you're after. Farther—not faster—is better.

In the beginning, you'll be doing interval training just like track athletes do. You must experiment to determine your appropriate walking and running intervals. It really doesn't matter whether your intervals are minutes, steps, sidewalk slabs, telephone poles, or city blocks. Eventually you'll be running more of them and walking less.

A word of caution on a different kind of pressing—for those of good endurance fitness but new to running. Your heart and lungs may be able to carry you three miles, but your joints and muscles might appreciate a mile and a half to start. In the course of a mile each foot strikes the ground about five hundred times. Once accustomed to it, your body takes this repetitive ground-stroke in stride. But when starting, let your body adapt slowly. Whatever you think you can run, cut it in half and try that distance. Your body will thank you with less stiffness and soreness, fewer aches and pains.

Pressing Later

Pressing in the beginning brings setbacks. Pressing later can be equally troublesome. *Run to Reality* offers the following advice for those who are fit but still choose to press:

> Enter each run
> in a way
> that allows
> the run
> to be formed
> from within.

When I start on a run I always have a rough idea of the direction in which I'll head and the amount of ground I'd like to cover. Body and spirit as my guide, I revel in a midrun change of course. Some fine days I go farther and faster than planned. This is where the "don't rush" persisting advice of Chapter Two comes in handy. An open-ended session allows the good runs to reach their natural conclusions.

Of greater importance is heeding the body when it says it wants to return home sooner than you planned. If you struggle on, you'll probably arrive home tired and not invigorated, and your risk of injury or soreness is increased.

I start my run a little slower than regular pace. Starting slower ensures comfortable aerobic running. With this approach I get the most—physically and philosophically—out of my run.

Technical Tips

Surfaces

Following the "pressing" issue of "how much to run" comes the question of surface or "where to run." The newspaper lady mentioned in Chapter One implied that one should run on sawdust or not at all. Fortunately, there's no evidence to suggest that there's any truth to what she says.

Sawdust trails, grass, dirt, firm gravel, and pavement (sidewalk or road) give a soft-to-hard hierarchy. If you choose only to run on sawdust trails, you limit your scenery. Trails around small city parks soon become as tedious as the nearby high-school track.

A better approach is to prepare yourself for any surface and thus not limit your horizon. As mentioned in Chapter One, this preparation includes a proper warmup, starting gradually, using a proper running style, and possessing shoes that adequately support the feet. I vie for proper preparation. This way, I go where the spirit moves me, not where the body dictates.

Dr. Kavanaugh suggests that road running offers no dangers. Better this, he says, than the risk of turning the ankle on uneven, but softer, ground. If you prefer softer turf, keep the surface hierarchy in mind. But remember: Grass, dirt, and gravel should be firm and flat or you increase your risk of ankle or knee strains.

Style

Entire books have been written about running style—something that is both a natural and an individual thing. The Foreword to *Running with Style* may have said all that's necessary. It suggests that running should be "individually fitted, speed adapted, mechanically efficient, and relaxed." Individually fitted means a natural and comfortable stride length. Overstriding can induce soreness and injury. Speed adapted implies a soft heel or flat-foot landing with a rock forward and *gentle* push off the toes. Being up on the toes like a sprinter or bouncing too much can lead to sore arches, calves, tendons, or shins. Mechanically efficient means an upright posture (not bent forward) and bent arms that move forward and back, not sideways across the chest. Arms are bent but elbows not locked; hands are loose but not flopping at the wrist. (Bill Bowerman suggests: "The elbows are bent slightly away from the body, neither out like wings nor pressed to the chest.") Relaxed? Well, *Running with Style* says, "Running with tension is like driving a car with the brakes on. You work harder to go slower."

Perhaps even this is more instruction than necessary. Percy Cerutty, a famous Australian distance running coach who into his seventies taught his athletes by example, said, "Watch children run and go and do likewise."

Shoes

Selection. A runner phoned one day to get some advice on new shoe purchase. He had read the latest shoe rankings in a running magazine and was in a quandary. He said he pounded a lot when he ran and now discovers his shoes are only ranked "twenty-third in heel shock absorption." It was then I knew some simplifying was called for.

The old reliable "tennies" are fine if you're going a mile or so each time, a few days a week. But if you run more ambitiously you'll need sturdier shoes that adequately support the feet, in turn protecting the knees, hips, and lower back. Many shoes fit the bill and all the good ones have some important qualities in common.

Your best first step is to find out where distance runners buy their shoes. These stores will carry a range of the better shoes and will likely have experienced sales attendants who can help you make a wise choice.

Keep the following in mind during your shoe search:

Shoes should be quite comfortable as soon as you put them on. "Break in" time should be minimal. Jog around the store in them if they'll let you (or even if they won't!).

The sole should be thick (.5 inch to 1 inch under the heel), offering good cushioning between you and the ground. To achieve this thickness, good shoes have a tough outer bottom layer followed by one or two softer layers. The sole should be solid but *flexible* under the ball of the foot for easy bending during the gentle pushoff with the toes.

The heel should be .5 inch to .75 inch higher than the toe. (The ideal difference, apparently, is 1.5 cm.). This elevation reduces strain on the lower leg (especially the Achilles tendon). Heel width is important, too, and moderation is the key. A heel too narrow may not give enough stability; whereas an extremely wide heel may hinder your natural running pattern and result in knee injuries.

The upper part of the better shoes are leather or nylon reinforced with leather (suede). The inside material should be nonirritating with few inside seams (they can cause rubbing). Nylon with leather uppers are soft yet supportive.

Look for shoes with a fitted leather layer around the back. This extra layer is known as a heel counter and, as its name implies, its job is to stabilize the heel. This heel counter should be quite rigid. The front of the shoe should have a wide, high toe box, roomy enough to avoid unnecessary rubbing on the toes and toenails. Finally, a leather layer, running around the top edge of the shoe, pads and supports the Achilles tendon, ankle, and instep.

Most shoes come in a standard width, but a few brands offer some variation. If you have an unusually wide or narrow foot, ask your local shoe experts which brands offer varying widths.

The day of the $9.95 running shoe is long gone, so be prepared to pay for quality. You may even need a couple of pairs a year depending on your running style, the kind of surface you run on, and your weekly mileage. This may seem quite a financial outlay, but figure the cost per mile and remember it's an investment in your health.

Finally, take no heed of shoe rankings once you've found shoes that are compatible. Why break up a winning combination?

Care and Repair. One friend, queried about his beat-up running shoes, said, "I've had them thirteen hundred miles." He also once said, "Those guys who run *super* long distances are crazy. I'd never run more than four hours without stopping." Ever since the "four hour" story I've been a little skeptical about the thirteen hundred miles.

However, good shoes do last a long time if you look after them. There was a time when worn-down soles meant the end of your shoes. No more. A variety of rubber glues are now available that allow you to build up worn-down heels and thus increase the life span of your "runners." All good running-shoe stores carry this ac- cessory. When your shoes have finally seen the end of their running days they're great for working in the garden. I know one person who took scissors to old shoes and ended up with blue nylon sandals.

It's common for the outside back part of the heel to wear first, as this is the natural landing spot. Keep an eye on them and build them back to level with the rest of the heel as they wear. An eighth inch or quarter inch of wear (at five hundred foot-strikes each mile) is enough to throw the foot out of its natural alignment and lead to injury problems (especially in the knee).

Running Attire

I offer two opposing views on running attire.

The first group are free spenders. They suggest you spoil yourself —go in luxury. Get a running outfit that feels good on your body and you feel good wearing. Get the best your budget allows. This purchase may help you persist when things get rough. You'll want to get your money's worth. Reward yourself with a big, fluffy towel after your bath or shower.

The conservative side says you don't get fitter faster if better dressed, so get into whatever is comfortable and get started. Old loose pants and a T-shirt are just fine. Perhaps later you can reward yourself for persisting with a new sweatsuit. This can come at a time when you know you're here to stay. One runner I know has worn the same outfit (regularly cleaned!) every session for the past 2½ years. His blue "Out-to-lunch Bunch" T-shirt is significantly faded, but his brown Bermuda shorts are no worse for the wear. He's now running farther but, as yet, has felt no compulsion to enhance his wardrobe. You decide the clothing philosophy that's right for you.

Weather permitting—shorts, T-shirt, socks, and shoes are all you need. A white cotton T-shirt may be best. Cotton is very absorbent, and white reflects heat the best. Light mesh tops are excellent in very hot weather. You may wish a brighter color for dusk or darkness running. Nylon shorts are the smoothest and minimize on chafing. Shoes already discussed, white sweatsocks (colored can leave dye on your feet) complete the picture.

If you face exceptionally cold or hot weather, it's important to take some sensible precautions. Obviously, shorts and a T-shirt won't be enough in the cold. The layered approach suggested for hikers is equally good for running, but important for a different reason. Layers in hiking allow you to adapt to changing conditions gradually. Layers in running mean you can be wet from sweat on the inside but still dry to the wind on the outside. A few layers to face the cold mean it'll take some time before you're wet right through.

The bottom layer should be absorbent and nonirritating (like our white T-shirt just mentioned). The next layer is for insulation. A cotton turtleneck offers warmth without weight. A hooded, pullover sweatshirt or a zippered sweattop serve quite well for the third layer. A fourth layer may be necessary for extremely cold or windy weather—a lightweight (for example, nylon) windbreaker here completes the upper-body attire. In very cold weather, a wool layer may be desired because of its warm-when-wet quality.

One layer on the legs should be sufficient for most conditions. (One prairie runner claims he only goes to two layers when the weather is below —100° F, including the wind-chill factor!) Long underwear and wool or nylon warmup pants all work well.

Accessories include a mask for the coldest weather and mittens (better than gloves). In both cases, wool is the best material for reasons previously mentioned.

Hot-weather running offers a whole different set of dangers. If you get into long-distance running or racing you may even search out information on temperature-humidity indices and wet-bulb globe temperatures. For those starting, it's enough to say—run a little slower in the heat, avoid the hottest part of the day (over 85° F. days you should plan an early-morning or evening run), and don't drastically increase your distance during hot spells. Increased fluid intake is important here, as it is in hot-weather hiking. See the Chapter Five information on electrolyte replacement drinks.

Injuries

Proper attention paid to preparation, pressing, surfaces, style, and shoes can mean less need to refer back to this section later. A wide range of problems await the runner who doesn't progress sensibly. As more people join the moving movement and the health of the nation improves, we may not need fewer doctors, but specialists of a different sort—more sports-medicine types and fewer cardiologists.

One last look at prevention before turning to common injuries.

Physicians specializing in sports medicine suggest that over half of the running injuries are due to faulty training practices—that is, too much, too soon. If one is to proceed wisely, running mileage should increase at a rate no faster than 10 per cent per week.

Injuries will be considered under common complaints, probable causes, and possible cures. Common complaints from beginners include shin splints; sore Achilles tendons and calves; sore arches and feet, and sore knees. I'll not encroach on the domain of the physician, physiotherapist, or podiatrist, but a few simple suggestions may help prevent or correct some small nagging problems. Problems that recur or persist require immediate professional advice.

Shin Splints. Pain along the inside border of the shinbone is a likely indicator you've got a case of shin splints. It can be a simple inflammation of the muscle along the edge of the bone or as serious as a straining or tearing of the muscle along the shin at the point where it attaches to the bone.

Going from no running to some running or changing from a soft to a hard surface may be enough to bring on this common ailment. Shoes with little shock absorption can magnify the problem. These are the likely causes for beginners. Muscles in the shin area that are weak or inflexible relative to the calf muscles and an improper foot plant can also be causal factors.

"Beginner" shin splints suggest running shorter distances at a slower pace for a few days to give your legs a chance to adapt to their newfound activity. More severe shin splints may require ice massage and a few days' rest. Proper shoes are mandatory! Transitory shin splints should subside with this care.

For persistent shin splints, medical advice will be necessary to determining whether foot structure, faulty foot plant, or weak muscles in the front of the shin are the root of your problem. One of the "magic six" exercises can look after weak shin muscles. Beyond this, your medical counselor is the one to suggest suitable corrective action.

Achilles Tendons and Calves. The calf muscle (gastrocnemius) and the long muscle (soleus) under it may rebel in the initial stages of running. Time spent on Exercises A-17 and 18 and B-17 can help avoid stiffness here. Shorter, slower distances or a little rest should be enough to rid you of this problem.

The Achilles tendon is a sensitive tendon that attaches the calf muscle to the heel bone. Problems here are potentially more troublesome than transitory sore calves. Tendonitis is evidenced by a tenderness to touch, swelling, or pain on walking or running. Don't be fooled if the pain subsides as you get into the run and are more warmed up. Quite likely the pain will return an hour or so after running when you've cooled down. Use these early warning signs to take steps to correct the problem, since this is one of the slowest-healing of injuries.

Tendonitis can result from building up your distance too quickly, running on hills too soon, inadequate shoes, or insufficient time spent on warmup suppleness exercises. Obvious preventive action, then, is progressing gradually, avoiding hills initially, well-heeled shoes, and religiously doing exercises A-18 and B-17. A more serious cause is faulty foot plant—landing on the outside edge of the foot *excessively* and then rolling inward. This last cause requires medical advice for correction.

If tendonitis develops, remedial procedures are crucial. Ice, rest, a heel lift for your shoes, and *patience* are the keys. Dr. Sheehan, writing for *Physician and Sports Medicine,* suggests that if tendonitis is caught within the first week, 95 per cent will be completely cured with two weeks of total rest. Of the remaining 5 per cent, half will be ready with another week of rest; the remainder will require up to six weeks of rest.

On the road to recovery, pain must be your guide. If it's not hurting you, you're probably not hurting it. Avoid stretching during the early rest-recovery stage. When running is possible, run at reduced pace and distances. Where possible run on smooth, flat surfaces and avoid sharp turns.

Persistent tendonitis may result from the above-mentioned foot imbalance and inward tilt on landing. As in persistent shin splints, medical advice should be sought.

Sore Arches and Feet. Blisters, nail pain, sore arches, and heel (stone) bruises can also greet the beginner. Two pairs of socks reduce rubbing, and new shoes should be broken in gradually (on shorter runs first, and alternated with old shoes). This should look after blisters. If they still visit, see the Chapter Five advice on blister care and repair. Nail pain is largely avoided by selecting shoes that are snug but not tight and tying them firmly enough that your feet don't slide forward in them on landing. The risk of sore heels is reduced by careful shoe selection (adequately thick heels and good arch supports) and proper running style (no pounding or *hard* heel landing). Sore arches can come from repeated flattening of the arch as the foot pronates (rolls inward) on landing. Arch exercises can help. "Toe pickups" (curling the toes under and picking up cotton batten), for example, and toe raises (standing and raising up on the toes) are good ones. Those with persistent problems may require a shoe insert to raise the heel and support the arch.

Sore Knees. Sore knees can be caused by your feet, your shoes, or the surface you run on. The most common of knee problems is *chondromalacia,* in medical terms—"runner's knee" to us. Runner's knee brings with it pain and tenderness under the kneecap or on either side of it. Pain results when the kneecap rides over the end of the thighbone instead of staying in the groove designed for it.

One common cause is an abnormal stress on the knee due to an incorrect foot plant. This can result from running on a slanted beach, on the shoulder of the road, around small flat tracks (like many indoor ones), or by wearing shoes with worn-down heels. (Worn-down heels accentuate the flattening of the long arch—or pronation—of the foot.) Again, obvious preventive procedures are to run on flat surfaces whenever possible, or in both directions on slanted ones and apply rubber "goo" early and liberally to worn-down shoes. Again, some people may require shoe inserts to correct a foot imbalance or faulty foot plant that leads to knee problems.

A second common cause of knee problems is insufficient quadricep (thigh) strength. Insufficient strength means that the knee joint is not adequately supported or protected. This concern appears more often in women than in men. Obvious methods to rectify the problem include some cycling or one of the telephone-book "magic six" exercises mentioned earlier in the chapter. If this is definitely your problem you may be wise to go beyond the telephone-book stage and invest in a pair of ankle weights. With them you can work to correct the deficiency, comfortably and easily over a period of time.

You can even start to improve the strength of very weak quadricep muscles by an action known as "quadricep setting." This is merely a contraction of the quadricep muscles while you're in a sitting position. Contract or "flex" the quadricep. Hold ten seconds. Do fifteen or twenty times a day. Remember to breathe normally—don't hold your breath—while you're doing this exercise.

"Jumper's knee" (*patellar tendonitis* in medical terms) is a further common injury most often brought on by excessive downhill running. Again, insufficient quadricep strength is one reason this problem occurs. As in most other injuries, a reduction in distance (or rest) and ice massage are imperative. Remedial quadricep strengthening exercises are then in order. Shoes with adequate support are crucial.

For persistent or serious problems, remember the Chapter Two advice on finding a sports-medicine physician. Let him decide if a physiotherapist or podiatrist ("foot doctor") can help you with some corrective exercises or shoe inserts. If you're lucky, you'll find a doctor who's a "one-stop shop"—someone who can tell you what's wrong, prescribe recovery procedures and, if worse comes to worst, even design shoe inserts. In this case no referral is necessary.

"Stitch." One further consideration is a "stitch." It's not an injury, more a minor irritation or short-term discomfort. This general term "stitch" is applied to a variety of pains experienced while exercising. The commonly accepted cause is lack of oxygen to the diaphragm due to improper breathing.

An extensive study at the University of Auckland summarized that most often "pain occurred during recurrent vertical jolting movements while the body is in an upright position." Running and sometimes cycling on a rough road can induce a stitch. The study noted that stitches were not common in swimmers or rowers.

Suggested methods to avoid a stitch include strengthening the stomach muscles (see Exercises 7, 8, and 10 of Series A and Series B), prerun stretching of the midsection (see Exercises A-2 and 3, B-2, 3, and 4), and avoiding food and liquid immediately before exercise.

If a stitch visits you in midrun, slow down or walk. "Belly" breathing, forcing the stomach out on inhalation and pulling it in on exhalation, can help. If necessary breathe deeply, bend forward, and press the hands on the painful area.

By now, you might be deleting running from your list of possible activities. Sounds like too many things can go wrong. However, the rewards far outweigh potential problems. Besides, the key is *prevention.* If you proceed wisely, you minimize the risk. In summary, choose shoes wisely, warm up properly, find the running surface that suits you best, increase your running distance gradually over a period of time, and, finally, react quickly to hints of pain. Don't wait until an injury is screaming out before you attend to it.

Safety

Be wary of cars when street crossing or if you run on the shoulder of a road. Wait for a generous break in the traffic before crossing. If you choose to sprint and dodge, you may say "Go," but tired legs say "No," and you're in trouble. If you must run on the shoulder of the road, run on the side facing oncoming traffic.

Be very visible if you like running at night. Bright clothing is imperative: Reflector tape is a bonus. If you're a lady runner concerned about running alone in some places or after dark, find a partner. Run with someone compatible who also offers a measure of protection.

The preceding advice is brief but sufficient for starters. It's aimed at the three-times-a-week beginner but can also help the seasoned runner maintain a sensible approach. Bad days and setbacks will be fewer if you heed the "pressing" information and the technical tips.

Even seasoned runners have bad and indifferent days. Sometimes you struggle along as though you've never run before. But as you progress they are fewer and farther between and it's the majority of positive runs that keep you coming back for more.

And then there are the special days—some that remain somehow, magically, in your mind. I've had my share of special runs, and for that I'll always be grateful.

Toronto, in mid-January, after a heavy snowfall is hidden somewhere deep inside me. I headed south toward the lake. Streetcars, usually slowed by traffic, were passing me with ease. The sharp blue of the sky and lake were a striking contrast to the white softness underfoot. I headed east along the boardwalk, breaking new tracks in the snow. I was alive with memories as I ran past a field, now vacant and snow-covered, where I played football five years before.

Nor am I likely to forget farm country of southwestern Ontario as winter turns to spring. It was definitely winter running, but there were thoughts of spring in the air. The sun was more generous with its warmth. Remnants of last fall's harvest were visible in fields of melting snow. I sensed that the farmers were readying for action. This back-road running brought farmhouses that were unique, clusters of trees that varied in size and shape, and a gentle rise and fall to the road. But always before me was a gravel road stretching as far as I could see. Sun and wind approaching from different angles were the only reminders that I had changed direction. Some would call this monotonous. Well, that's up to them, I guess. To me it had a certain vastness and it brought with it a wonderful sense of freedom.

But, for me, beach running is the best, and Henry's Beach in Santa Barbara is where I always wish to return. Cliffs protect and catch gentle breezes off the ocean. I look up or down the beach from where I always start, and the cliff, the sand, and the water join on the distant horizon. The beach is wide, flat, hard-packed, and endless. I like the endless part best. And the ocean? Its power fills you and leaves a feeling both difficult to understand and impossible to forget.

One late afternoon in May I ran on this beach, first northwest into the sun. I remember seeing a dark-brown, cliffside house partially hidden by trees. I'd run here every day for a week. Funny I hadn't seen it before. Other than this, I didn't see or think much; I just felt the run.

With much heat and little wind, it was a day for just shorts and shoes. First, sweat broke on my forehead, then my chest and shoulders. Soon I was dripping wet—a product of the sun, the heat, and the motion. I ran as far as high tide would allow, then returned with the sun at my back.

At run's end I was greeted by a friend I had met here at the beach earlier in the week. Tom was retired and he wandered yearly, west from Arizona to the coast, north to Canada, and back home down through the mountains. He met me, offered a cold beer, and we sat on a picnic table and talked. His dark tan and sprightly stride were testimony to his long daily walks on the beach. We shared this beach and, I think, knew it in a different way than did the bathers and surfers.

I'll always remember these runs, but, even better, I know I can expect many more like them in the years to come. I also know that you can't strive for or work toward them. They just happen. They sneak up on you at the most unexpected times and in some beautiful places. And though these runs are unique, they share a common thread, and a comfortable feeling that's easily understood but difficult to explain to others. Ron Clarke, renowned Australian distance runner, once spoke of weekly mileage common only to athletes, but of this feeling we all can capture.

. . . and still I cannot define precisely my joy in running. There is no sacrifice in it. I lead what I regard a normal life. . . . I could not imagine a life devoid of some form of physical exercise and, in my case, I thoroughly enjoy running one hundred-odd miles a week. If I didn't, I wouldn't do it. Who can define happiness? . . . To me, happiness is running in the hills with my mates around me.

This inability to define the exact meaning of running is, perhaps, part of its intrigue. Some days it's just a need for movement—a time to get away from it all or solve it all. Other days it's simply one carefree step after another, returning when the time seems right, remembering not where or how far you went but only how good it felt every step of the way. Then those special days, the ones that leave you with, "I've never ever felt quite like this before."

Out of all this, a last piece of advice for beginners: Keep an open mind. Run for fitness, but contemplate the possibility of something greater. George Sheehan says running for fitness "is like taking up painting to improve the strength of your arm." It's not just a physical thing. It's mental and physical, therapy and ecstasy. Rob Inman, practicing physician and dear friend, wrote:

The close relation of mind and body is something you see on the wards every day. But even in health there are degrees of that unity. The joy of running is a step toward that.

B. C. Runner (quarterly)
Seawall Running Society
P.O. Box 4981
Vancouver, B.C., Canada V6B 4A6

The Runner (monthly)
New Times Publishing Company
One Park Avenue
New York, N.Y. 10016

Fixx, James F. *The Complete Book of Running*.
New York: Random House (1977), 314 pp.

Henderson, Joe. *Thoughts on the Run*.
Mountain View, Calif.: World Publications (1970), 109 pp.

Rohé, Fred. *The Zen of Running*.
New York: Random House; Berkeley, Calif.: The Bookworks (1974).

Sheehan, George A. *Dr. Sheehan on Running.*
New York: Bantam (1978), 205 pp.

——. *Running and Being: The Total Experience.*
New York: Simon and Schuster (1978), 256 pp.

CHAPTER SEVEN

I'm Not Quite There Yet

CYCLING

BIKE SELECTION
Number of Speeds
Size, Weight, and Cost
Saddle and Handlebars
Brakes, Wheels, and Tires
Used Bikes
Accessories

SETUP, MAINTENACE, AND REPAIR

FITNESS RIDING
Starting
Progressing
Injuries

COMMUTING AND TOURING
Clothing
Equipment
Safety
Locking
Transporting
Riding Style
Hot-weather Riding

Biking is freedom—freedom from the city, from your cares, from the humdrum. It invigorates and brings you in touch with what's happening around you and in tune with nature. Experience the romantic changes of the day—a crisp dawn, a sunny noon, a starry night. Feel the breezes, taste the salt spray off the ocean, touch a redwood. Enjoy the best things about being alive.

—Sue Browder
American Biking Atlas and Touring Guide

IN OUR urbanized, fast-moving world, bicycling may not be a panacea, but it's about as close as you can come. As a fitness activity, it's one of the best. As low-cost, practical transportation, it's hard to beat, and for the sheer joy of getting out and moving, well, just listen to the hard-core cyclists. They're as fanatical as runners in extolling the virtues of their activity.

At the financial level, a new bicycle is about one fortieth the cost of a new car. A bicycle runs almost maintenance-free from one year to the next. If you're a two-car family, I leave it to you to calculate the savings if one family member could turn to regular cycle commuting. In your calculation, remember to consider your (tax-free) capital gain from the sale of your car along with adding your expected yearly savings in gas, parking, new tires, parts, maintenance, and repair. One film on bikeways suggested that 60 per cent of all urban commuting trips cover five miles or less. To any moderately fit cyclist this is leisurely accomplished in less than half an hour—not much more time than a car requires in normal city traffic.

A return to "pedal power" is a move in the right direction in a time when energy sources are dwindling and becoming more expensive. The bicycle is nonpolluting, human-powered, and occupies little space. (You can park ten bikes in the area filled by one car.) Just as improved health on the part of each individual (by choosing healthful lifestyle habits) can help slow the staggering growth in health-care costs, increased bicycle usage could slow the need for costly highway development in urban areas.

Cycling is a change in lifestyle and, in turn, can lead to a changed way of thinking. For motorists, rain means slow traffic and a dash from car to cover. To the cyclist who is careful and watches the traffic, rain can be one element contributing to a special day. Cyclists, of all people, know that fastest is not necessarily best.

Dr. Irvine H. Page, onetime president of the American Heart Association, was attributed with a statement that nicely sums up the situation:

> We ought to replace the automobile with bicycles. . . . It would be better for our coronaries, our dispositions, and certainly our finances.

In spite of all its advantages, a mass move to bicycles won't happen overnight. It'll take time to change a nation's way of thinking. Converting a generation brought up on the automobile, the elevator, and television will be no easy task. However, if you're looking for a change and cycling's a possibility, the following information—from bike selection through tips for commuting and touring—aims to help you start properly.

Bike Selection

The first and obvious suggestion is to shop around. Make the rounds of the bike shops and get a feel for the market. Talk to the guys who do repairs. They know good from bad. They fix them all day long.

Don't make a rash decision. You wouldn't hastily buy a new car, would you? See if you can borrow some bikes for trial rides. Keep the following in mind as you shop:

Number of Speeds

Four main types are available. First comes the child's fun bike (perhaps out of the question for most readers). Next up the line is the one-gear, usually a heavyweight, the bike of our youth for those of us over twenty-five. It's the old model with balloon tires and pedal brakes, long ago discarded but likely still operational somewhere.

Next comes the middleweight three-gear, known as a standard when I was young. It's less common now but still suitable for local shopping trips and leisurely rides around the neighborhood.

Now dominating the market are five- and ten-gear touring bikes.

The five-gear is quite sufficient for weekend rides and almost all commuting. (It's lighter than a three-speed, and five gears make it easier to pedal and more versatile.)

Commuting in cities like San Francisco, Montreal, and Vancouver, and longer touring may require more gears. The ten-gear is the logical answer. It's slightly more expensive than the five-gear, but it greatly increases gear ratios and allows for comfortable pedaling over a wide variety of terrain.

Size, Weight, and Cost

The salesperson can help you pick the right size. Some measure by having you straddle the bike (looking for about half an inch between your crotch and the top bar); others may measure your inseam length and deduct ten inches to arrive at frame size.

If you're less than five feet tall, don't despair! Some bicycle manufacturers offer adult bikes in smaller than standard frames.

Thirty-five to thirty-eight pounds is common for a five-gear bike, twenty-seven or thirty-three pounds for a ten-gear bike. Lighter bikes (for racing and touring) cost more. (You pay more to get less.) Good bikes are constructed as light as possible without sacrificing structural strength and safety. (A noted bicycle designer once said that the only place weight is desired is in a steamroller.)

One comment on costs: Avoid the $59.95 variety. Quality is low, and potential repair costs are high. Bike shops carry a wide variety of good bikes of both domestic and foreign origin. Choose something of good quality that also suits your budget.

Saddle and Handlebars

A plastic saddle is standard issue on five- and ten-gear bikes. It's a practical saddle and weather-resistant. Leather saddles need only be considered if you're covering more than twenty-five miles a day. Leather stays cooler than plastic, and in time (like a good running shoe that forms to your foot) it forms to the shape of *your* seat.

The wide, soft, comfortable-looking saddle is common on single-, three-, and five-gear bikes. It's fine for around-town cycling and short trips. The ten-gear comes with a narrower, longer saddle. It's more comfortable and allows more efficient cycling on longer rides.

Five-gear and lesser-gear bikes usually have upright handlebars, whereas drop bars are standard on ten-gear bikes. The drop-style bars are important for longer rides. They allow a variety of hand-arm-upper-body positions. A forward-leaning position, with much of the weight supported by the hands and arms, takes pressure off the lower back.

Brakes, Wheels, and Tires

Many of the reasonably priced ten-gear bikes include safety levers. These are a second set of brake levers on the crosspiece of the handlebar. They permit more convenient braking when sitting in the upright position, since the standard brake levers are on the down part of the handlebar. In the interest of safety, these extra levers are wisely avoided. First, they can't be used if you have a handlebar bag. Second, and more important, they reduce the distance your brake levers can travel before hitting the handlebars, thus compromising braking action.

New multispeed bikes in the lower price categories almost always come with chrome-plated steel wheels. These are quite sufficient but later on some serious cyclists substitute the less durable aluminum-alloy type. They don't tolerate rough treatment as well but they offer measurably better braking action under *all* weather conditions.

Two choices exist in the tire line: tubular or clincher. Tubular tires are more vulnerable to puncture, they weigh less, and they are easy to change. They're the favorite of racers and long-distance riders. The clincher or "wire-on" is the conventional type. The inner tube, once inflated, forces the outer cover against the sides of the rim in a snug fit. They're more difficult to change, but are better for most bicycle needs, and are standard on ten-gear bikes. Racers must buy special rims for their tubular tires.

Used Bikes

Newspaper ads and communal bulletin boards in laundromats, stores, and college dorms are your first stops in search of a used bike.

Check for rust, examine the frame for damage, search for missing parts, and look and *listen* as you change gears and spin wheels. Bike shops often give some kind of a guarantee (usually for thirty days). No guarantee on private deals means they're a little more risky.

Expect to pay half to three quarters of new bike price. Weigh the asking price and repair and replacement costs against the cost of a new one.

Accessories

If you're just starting to ride, buy the least possible equipment and add items as you find they're needed. Head- and taillights and reflectors; fenders (if you're an all-weather rider); a tire pump; and toe clips and straps are rightly called necessities, not accessories. Beyond these items, hesitate before you buy anything more.

Front (white) and rear (red) lights and rotating reflectors that attach to the spokes (orange for the front and red for the back) are mandatory after dark. Front and rear lights should be visible from five hundred feet. Wheel- and battery-generated lights are both acceptable; however, wheel-powered lights may prove less desirable since riding speed determines light brightness.

An additional recommended item is a French light. You attach it by means of a strap, below your left knee or above your right elbow. It has lights facing front and rear and its motion increases your visibility.

Fenders are not standard on all bikes but prove valuable in inclement weather. They can reduce the need for a postride change of clothes.

Toe clips and straps are the final "necessary accessories." These are light metal loops that extend up over the toes of your shoes from the front edge of the pedals. Straps run from the inside to the outside of the pedal across your instep. They help maintain correct positioning of the feet on the pedals and they assist in "ankling," allowing a pull as well as a push on the pedal. They should be worn loosely for quick withdrawal of the foot in city riding, tighter for extended touring.

Setup, Maintenance, and Repair

Attention paid to proper setup and regular maintenance will result in fewer breakdowns and less need of repair. Weighed against repair, maintenance is less time-consuming and is cheaper. Full details on setup, maintenance, and repair are beyond the scope of this book. Following a good maintenance manual brings a systematic approach, whereas fiddling, if you're unfamiliar with the workings of a bike, can bring more problems than it solves. The recognized leading books on bike care and repair are *Delong's Guide to Bicycles and Bicycling* and Tom Cuthbertson's *Anybody's Bike Book*. Consider either a necessity.

Saddle height and angle deserve brief consideration. The disadvantages of a saddle too low or too high were described in Chapter Four. Too low means the thigh muscles tire more quickly, and too high has you rolling side to side over the seat to reach the pedals. The rolling motion means uncomfortable and less efficient pedaling.

The surface of the saddle should be horizontal (that is, no saddle angle). A saddle tilting down at the front causes you to slide forward, requiring you to push slightly with your arms to keep you back on the saddle. The result is early tiring of the arms, upper back, shoulders, and neck. A saddle tilting up causes an extreme tilt of the pelvis and undue fatigue (and possibly strain) on the lower back.

An understanding of one's bike and time spent fine-tuning can be part of the sport's fascination. Tom Cuthbertson, discussing the rewriting of his book to better co-ordinate the illustrations and text, said, "There's a dance that goes on between reading, seeing a picture, and looking at the bike. I'd like to improve the rhythm of that dance."

One final piece of advice from a *Bicycling* magazine article on maintenance:

> Work on your bike when you're feeling good. If four cups of coffee or other frustrations are upon you, don't take it out on your bicycle.

As your interest and knowledge grow, you can decide how much you wish to tackle yourself and how much you'll hand over to the expert at the repair shop.

Fitness Riding

Starting

If you're a real beginner, in fitness *and* cycling, take it easy. Avoid big hills at first. Don't venture off to school or to work until you're ready for it. Severe breathlessness or tired and sore legs mean you're building up too quickly. Use your target heart rate as a guide. Three or four days a week a few minutes each day are enough at the beginning. The "magic" fifteen minutes is as relevant here as it is in indoor cycling or running. And once again; remember your warmup and some cooldown exercises.

Progressing

As your fitness improves, don't fool yourself and coast. The multi-gear bike was a great invention but it can make cycling a breeze. Fifteen minutes of nonstop running may be out of the question for most people when starting, but just about everyone can pedal fifteen. Slow cycling requires little effort.

Heart rate counting is usually a reminder not to overdo it. You can use it here to good advantage to make sure you're not "underdoing" it. If the ride seems too easy, stop, count, and see if it's too slow to develop that precious training effect.

Cycle commuting is a different matter. The fifteen-minute idea is irrelevant, since you leave home with a specific destination. If you live ten miles from work and don't cycle now (and drive-cycle commuting isn't possible), don't start riding to work immediately. (At twenty miles a day, that's a hundred miles a week!) Build up gradually. Ride around the block and around the neighborhood, and go on evening and Saturday rides to prepare for the daily twenty-mile round trip.

If you're like me and live fairly close to work, riding's great for transportation but doesn't do much for your fitness. As you progress, ride a more circuitous route home—add some miles and ride harder. Stretch the leg muscles before your ride and then do your series of stretching and strengthening exercises at home following your longer return trip.

When moving from commuting to touring, the same "make haste slowly" principle applies. A veteran cyclist warns, "For heaven's sake, don't go and ride a thirty-five-mile day right away. Go five miles a day for a while, then ten, then fifteen. . . . Break in gradually. It might be two or three months before you're ready for a thirty-five-mile ride."

"Or six months?" I say.

"Or six months if you're really starting from the beginning."

Legs must grow "cycling fit" and your seat must get accustomed to sitting on the saddle for longer and longer periods of time.

In the end there's no magic way to increase other than slowly, gradually, patiently. One cyclist complained to a bicycle magazine about their overabundance of information on how to train for racing. Every month they offered something new—endurance; speed; concentration on spin; LSD or no LSD. He was confused. Eddy Merckx, a Belgian cyclist, many time winner of the Tour de France and one of the few cyclists ever conferred with the title *campionissimo* (champion of champions), has an answer for this confusion. Once queried on the strategy of his training program, he answered, "Ride lots." The same holds true for the recreational rider. Build up gradually, then "ride lots." It's as simple as that.

Injuries

My cycling guru, a wealth of information, said, "There are no common injuries." One reason is that as a weight-supported activity, pounding and jolting are minimal. There are, in fact, a few injuries particular to riding, but they are usually less severe and visit less often than do running injuries. The lower back, knees, and ankles are susceptible to problems. Proper setup and bike maintenance can help here.

A horizontal saddle (reducing stress on the lower back) and a saddle height that allows a slight bend of the knee are important. In addition, make sure your feet point straight ahead. Toeing in or out, putting unnatural stresses on the knee, can prove troublesome on long rides. The knees are the most vulnerable part of the body to cycling injuries and, as in running, it's the long-distance people who are most susceptible to problems. A suggested remedy for sore knees is a reduction in distance or, if necessary, taking some time off. While riding with sore knees, keep them warm, gear low, hills to a minimum, and don't fight pain. Important preventive stretching exercises for cycling are A-5, 6, 15, 17, and 18, and B-5, 6, 11, 15, 17, and 18. Remember they can (and should!) be done regularly for warmup and postride cooldown.

If pain persists, see your doctor (a sports-medicine type, if you can, as suggested in Chapter Two). Where I once lived, all the swimmers took their infections to one doctor, the runners their sore legs to another. You might even find a "bicycling doctor" where you live.

Cuts and abrasions are final considerations. Deal with them immediately to avoid infection. Keep them clean and covered with a clean dressing until dry, and then leave them open.

Commuting and Touring

Commuting (utility riding) and touring (recreational riding) require further considerations.

Clothing

Cyclists are wise to follow the layered approach suggested earlier for hikers and runners. You can strip off layers as you or the day warm up. As previously mentioned, avoid rubberized tops or suits, which can dangerously increase body temperature. Jeans and other pants with ridged inseams should be avoided, since they can cause chafing and blisters. Shirts should be light-colored for sunny riding, brightly colored or fluorescent for night rides. Cotton socks and solid shoes that firmly support the feet are best. A hard-soled shoe distributes pressure from the pedal throughout the entire foot, thus reducing fatigue. Cycling shoes are standard for racers and long-distance touring types. You might consider them if you progress to long-distance riding.

Hats, helmets, sunglasses, and gloves, often considered accessories, are worth contemplating as necessities. Cycling gloves are usually open-fingered, double-palmed leather and are cool to wear because of the loose weave on top. The layers of leather between you and your handlebars help reduce both pressure on your palms and grip slippage (since the leather absorbs sweat). Finally, gloves protect from "road rash" if you fall.

A hat, sunscreen, and sunglasses give protection on longer trips. Beware of sunburn—the cooling headwind of riding masks effects of the sun. Sunglasses are important, commuting or touring, as eye protection. A bug in the eye at twenty miles an hour is painful and can cause serious injury.

Few commuters wear helmets, but they're worth serious consideration. Helmets are standard on motorcycling. Landing impact from a fall at twenty miles an hour is the same whether you're on a bike or on a motorcycle. Two cycling helmets generally available are far superior to all the other brands. Ask your local experts what type to look for.

Equipment

Saddlebags (panniers) that fit astride the rear wheel are best for carrying heavy equipment. They distribute the weight evenly and low. If panniers are not sufficient, handlebar bags are useful for extra equipment. Keep the load light—otherwise it can affect your steering abilities. (Some cyclists prefer handlebar bags or a back-pack for shorter trips. A jacket and lunch fit here conveniently.)

Additional equipment you'll probably need if you get into longer touring include a water bottle, first-aid supplies, and some dog repellent.

Safety

The commuter on city streets faces more hazards than the touring cyclist on the open highway. Right-turning cars that cross your path, as well as opening car doors are obvious hazards. Expect the worst, be ready for it, and you're on your way to safe city riding. Obey *all* traffic rules, signal turns, be courteous to motorists, and they'll *probably* reciprocate.

Donald Pruden, in *Around Town Cycling*, offers wise advice to commuters:

● Reconnoiter alternative routes. Pick the one with the fewest potential traffic hassles.

● Travel the routes at different times. Five minutes earlier or later may greatly affect traffic density.

● Once settled on a route, travel the same time each day. You'll encounter the same people and they'll begin to anticipate your presence.

In a nutshell, Pruden offers four tips for survival in a car's world:

Be aware.
Be defensive.
Be predictable.
Be visible.

Locking

Theft prevention is virtually impossible. The best you can hope to do is provide the prospective thief with poor conditions for a fast, safe getaway.

Use a heavy, case-hardened chain or steel cable (covered in plastic) and lock. The cable should be no less than three-eighths inch in diameter. Make sure the chain length allows you to thread it through both wheels, around the frame, and around an immovable object like a tree or a telephone pole.

Leave your bike unattended as little as possible. Take it inside whenever you can. If you have quick-release wheels, take the front wheel with you.

If you can't wheel it inside stores or restaurants, park it right in front where it's easy to keep an eye on. When parking in a public area with other bikes, park near a more expensive one.

As for recovering your bike after a theft, recording and filing the serial number is a good start. If licensing or registration is available in your area, take advantage of it. It won't guarantee that your bike will be returned, but it'll increase the odds in your favor.

Transporting

If you can't ride all the way to your commuting destination, consider a drive-ride combination. Commuting to work this way may allow you to park free in a residential area and complete the trip by bike. In this case, you may need a bike carrier for your car. Good bumper carriers are solidly constructed and have rubber-covered hanger hooks, which reduce chipping and scratching of your bike. Cheaper racks rust easily, are unsturdy, and scratch your bike more often.

If you're carrying your bike long distances inside the car or in the trunk, you may want to remove the pedals, loosen the handlebar, and turn it ninety degrees so it's parallel with the frame (retighten in this position), remove quick-release wheels, and protect the *derailleur* with a cloth or some newspaper.

Riding Style

Riding style is not a concern on short trips but is increasingly important as the ride lengthens. Proper seat setup and toe clips allow "ankling"—use of the ankle joint. This technique gives power beyond that possible in a strict downward pushing motion using only the hips and the knees. A drop of the heel when the pedal is at the top allows a forward as well as a downward push. Dropping the toe at the bottom of the pedal action permits a backward and then upward pull. Proper "ankling" increases effective pedaling range from a maximum of 170° to anywhere between 270° and 310°, depending on the refinement of technique. Exercises A-17 and A-18 will help prepare your lower legs for this "ankling" action.

Proper pedaling cadence or frequency is another important factor. The motive for gear change is a *constant* and comfortable pedaling cadence. Don't pedal slowly uphill and fast down, slowly into the wind and fast with it behind you. Change gears for smooth pedaling regardless of terrain or wind conditions. A beginner should aim for 60 to 70 revolutions per minute. Veteran riders and racers may be in the 90-to-100 range. On long rides they may start at 90 to 100 and drop the rate later in the day as fatigue builds. Experiment and find the frequency for you. Gear down on the inclines so tired thighs don't limit you. Take advantage of whatever number of gears you paid for. Don't apply power—pedal lightly forward (and never backward)—as you change gears.

Sitting too upright is tiring and offers greater resistance into the wind. A comfortable forward lean helps distribute the weight more evenly over the saddle, the handlebars, and the pedals. For faster speeds or strong headwinds, a lower, more streamlined position is appropriate.

Hot-weather Riding

Consider the Chapters Five and Six advice to hikers and runners about activity in hot weather. Adapt to hot-weather riding gradually and avoid the hottest part of the day at first. Drink proper kinds of fluids at regular intervals as mentioned in Chapter Five. Dress lightly in "air breathing" material in the heat.

Cycling, like all other fitness activities, can bring that difficult starting and persisting period. I faced it one summer when an injury left me with pain even on a slow jog. Advised to avoid running for a while, I turned to cycling to stay in shape.

It was strange to leave running, where I felt strong and confident, turn to cycling, and feel a beginner again. These two activities involve different muscle groups, so as a newcomer to cycling I had to be patient and build up slowly, allowing my muscles to adapt. As I was becoming "cycling fit," I had my share of bad and indifferent days. I was in the persisting phase where only a purpose, a destination could keep me going. I'd usually set off with a goal in mind. I'd ride a longer route to work, ride to my parents' place, or to the university. I needed a goal to motivate me, an outlook so different from my running. My runs had meaning. I needed a purpose in my cycling.

But one day I broke through. For the first time there was a certain ease and exhilaration in the ride. I was learning to maintain my pedaling speed. I was shifting gears sooner (making the hills less awesome), and my legs were getting stronger. I knew I wasn't quite there yet, but I was definitely on my way. And for the first time I *really* understood that the road that cyclists travel is much the same as the runner's.

Many runners start for fitness and finally just run to run. Some cyclists start commuting (fitness being a valuable by-product) and end up touring. In either case, many find a strange attachment, a new feeling, and a new attitude toward their activity.

Donald Pruden offers:

> Utility cycling—riding a bike because it's practical—leads to the harder stuff; not because of some bittersweet masochistic incentive, but because riding regularly taps unique, long-lost body-mind pleasures.

Longer rides bring the same opportunities as daily runs. It's a temporary exodus from day-to-day activities—a kind of suspended animation. A good friend and coworker rides many miles as he makes his rounds from home to school and work. I always envied him those rides—the speed, the ease of it, and the momentary freedom. After the day I broke through on my bike I surely knew that he gets the same from his ride as I capture on my run.

Touring and country camping bring even more. The ride itself, offers new sights, sounds, and smells, or familiar and cherished ones. Day's end can mean lounging on a sleeping bag, tea in hand, in front of an open fire. The ride brings a satisfying tiredness, and the relaxation after is a luxury hard to surpass. One comes to learn that a body well treated and properly conditioned performs remarkably. But even more than this, there's a sense of pride to know that you covered the day's distance self-propelled, unaided by man's modern inventions.

Runners may be more vocal and prolific than cyclists, but given the chance, cyclists refuse to let you believe that transcendence is solely a running phenomenon. One cyclist, in a testimony to the District of Columbia City Council concerning regulations for bicycling, was moved to say:

> The air feels good on your body. You hear things and smell things you never knew were there. The blood starts moving around and pretty soon it gets to your head and, glory be, your head feels good. You start whistling original tunes to suit the moment, and words start getting caught in the web of poetry in your mind.

Bicycling (monthly)
C. M. Publications
P.O. Box 4450
San Rafael, Calif. 94903

Cuthbertson, Tom. *Anybody's Bike Book.*
Berkeley, Calif.: Ten Speed Press (1977), 178 pp.

Delong, Fred. *Delong's Guide to Bicycles and Bicycling.*
London: Chilton's (1974), 278 pp.

TOURING INFORMATION

Bicycle Institute of America, Inc.
122 East 42nd Street
New York, N.Y. 10017

Canadian Cycling Association
333 River Road
Vanier City, Ont., Canada K1L 8B9

League of American Wheelmen
19 South Bothwell
Palatine, Ill. 60067

CHAPTER EIGHT

The Silent World

SWIMMING

WATER EXERCISE
The Exercises
Techniques

SERIES S EXERCISES

SWIM PROGRESSION
F—Frequency
I—Intensity
T—Time
T—Type
"Swimdown"—Cooldown

OTHER MATTERS
Bathing Suits
Goggles and Plugs
Injuries
Safety

What a piece of work is a man! . . .
in form and moving how express and admirable!
in action how like an angel!
—*Hamlet*, II, ii, 317

WE ALL have our biases. One swimming instructor said his activity
was the best, the most accessible because all you needed was a
bathing suit. I thought, "It's not quite that easy; you need some
water too." Admittedly, I have my favorite. But there are many an-
swers, and swimming—as a vehicle for health and fitness—ranks
with the best of them.

Water has a dual personality. Its buoyancy and support soften
the infirmities of advancing age, allowing graceful and gentle
movement. Move with greater force and the water resists. Buoyancy and support, yet resistance? A pleasant and helpful contradiction.

The water has something for everyone. It's an ideal medium for
those with back problems, arthritis, and other joint disorders. Physiotherapists have long used it for retraining and rehabilitation from
injury, illness, and accident. For fitness, swimming brings a balanced development—upper and lower body strength and suppleness—that no other single activity can match. And for fun there's
skin and scuba diving, synchronized swimming, water polo (for the
skillful), and inner-tube water polo (for the playful).

Just about everyone has a chance to swim. Our swim instructor
really wasn't far off when he said your only need is a bathing suit.
The necessary "water" is daily more abundant. A pool is an integral
part of all newly constructed recreation complexes. One-upmanship
in urban housing means that a pool and an exercise area are no
longer frills but expected features in condominium and apartment
developments. If down the hall or down the elevator leads to a
pool, then swimming is as accessible as walking, running, or cycling. It's one more option—another possibility, and, perhaps, the
one that proves right for you.

Travelers with a skipping rope and exercise charts have their
gymnasium in a suitcase. If you're a swimmer, search out accommodations with a pool. Pack a bathing suit and you're ready for action.

Water Exercise

Hydrotherapy—active or passive movements while partially or completely submerged in warm water—is a popular and effective rehabilitation procedure. Some muscle and bone injuries, strained and torn ligaments, nerve and muscle diseases, psychogenic paralysis, paraplegia, and other problems respond to this kind of treatment.

Physical educators figured that if the exercises helped make sick people better, why not use them to keep healthy people healthy? Some were not satisfied with the simplicity of the term "water exercise," and new names flourished—"swim-nastics," "aquabics," and "aquasize" among them. By any name, they're exercises done in the water.

The elderly, the less fit, and the less skilled swimmer can all gain from them. They bring two of the three s's—suppleness and strength—and so are useful if you're not yet efficient in the water. Regardless of skill and fitness levels, they serve as excellent warmup routines to swimming.

The Exercises

Many land exercises are directly transferable to the water. Eleven of the Series A and Series B exercises (A-1, 2, 3, 4, 15, 16, 17, and 18, and B-4, 14, and 18) as outlined in Chapter Three are appropriate. They are all gentle-movement or stretch-and-hold suppleness exercises. As you progress do more repetition of the gentle-movement type, and "hold" the stretch-and-hold ones for a longer period of time. Refer to Chapter Three sketches and descriptions to ensure that you do them properly.

Remember, if you move more quickly, the water resists. Exercises A-1, 3, and 4, and B-4 can, therefore, double as strengtheners. The speed at which you do them will determine whether they primarily stretch or strengthen. A little of both kind is probably the best approach.

But this picking and choosing from Series A and Series B and flipping back to Chapter Three may seem a little haphazard. If so, a tight, self-sufficient series of seven water exercises follows. Consider it Series S. Series A, then Series B implied a certain progression. Calling this one Series C would, therefore, be inappropriate, since these exercises are done in the water and they stand alone as different from A and B. Call it Series S for swimming.

The following chart outlines the name and number of the exercise, the type (suppleness or strength), and the body part exercised. The seven exercises are really eleven, since S-1 and S-7 each have three parts.

WATER EXERCISES
SERIES S

Exercise Number and Name	Type of Exercise	Body Part Exercised
1. Upper Rotators (wrists, elbows and shoulders)	suppleness	arms and shoulders
2. Knee-Ups 3. Leg Crossovers	strength	stomach, trunk and hips
4. Flutter Kicking	strength	stomach, trunk, hips and legs
5. Toe Bouncing 6. Split Bouncing	strength	legs
7. Lower Rotators (ankles, knees and hips)	suppleness	legs

Techniques

As in Chapter Three, the exercise sketch is accompanied by a description explaining the starting position, the action, the nature of the exercise, and special points to watch for. A reminder for the strenghtening exercises: No breath holding, and exhale on effort, for the reasons mentioned in Chapter Three.

For the standing exercises (S-1, 5, 6, and 7), chest-deep water is best. Squat slightly, if necessary, to keep the shoulders and arms submerged. If you tend to lose your balance, do the exercises near the poolside and hold the deck or gutter with one hand for support. Exercises S-2, 3, and 4 are done holding the poolside or gutter with the hands and with the feet not touching the bottom.

As in the land-based exercises, don't rush. Learn the correct technique from the very beginning. If you tend to forget the exercises, jot them down on a card, add rough sketches, cover the card with plastic, and take it along with you to the pool.

If you find water exercises useful and enjoyable you may find the appropriate Series A and Series B exercises and Series S not enough to keep you busy and happy. If so, Sidney Shapiro's *Swim-nastics* and *Aqua Dynamics* from the President's Council on Physical Fitness and Sports both offer well-organized and complete series of exercises. Either booklet is an excellent investment.

Series S Exercises

1. **Upper rotators**
(wrists, elbows, and shoulders)

2. **Knee-ups**

3. **Leg crossovers**

4. **Flutter kicking**

5. **Toe bouncing**

6. **Split bouncing**

7. **Lower rotators**
(ankles, knees, and hips)

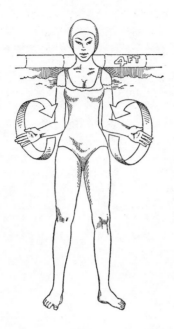

S-1
UPPER ROTATORS

Best done in wrist, elbow, shoulder order.

Elbow Rotators

Starting Position: Standing, arms bent at the elbows, elbows near your sides, hands in front.

Action: Slow, sweeping circles with the lower arm, keeping elbows at your sides. Circle inward, rest, repeat circling outward.

Nature of Exercise: Gentle, continuous, circular motion.

Important Points: Large, slow circles, not small, fast ones.

Wrist rotators and *shoulder rotators* (see A-1) are accomplished the same way with rotation around the appropriate joint.

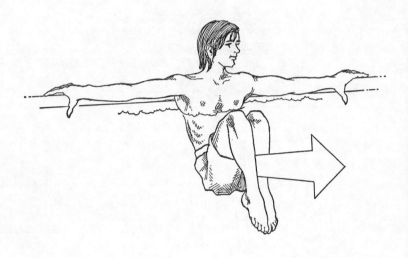

S-2
KNEE-UPS

Back to the poolside, arms outstretched holding the gutter or edge of the deck, legs straight in front, floating near the surface.

Bend at the knees and hips, dropping the seat down. Pull the knees in toward the chest. Return to straight position. Repeat.

Gentle, continuous, in-and-out (stretch-and-tuck) movement.

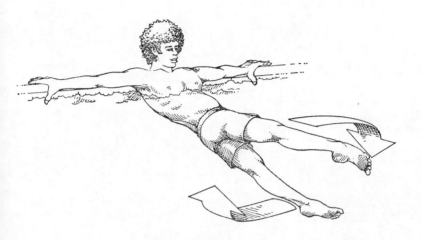

S-3
LEG CROSSOVERS

Back to the poolside, arms outstretched, holding the gutter or edge of the pool, legs straight in front, floating near the surface (same position as for S-2).

Spread the legs, then pull them together allowing the right hip to tilt up toward the surface and the right leg to cross *over* the left. Spread them again, then roll the left hip toward the surface and cross the left leg *over* right.

Gentle, side-to-side, crossover movement.

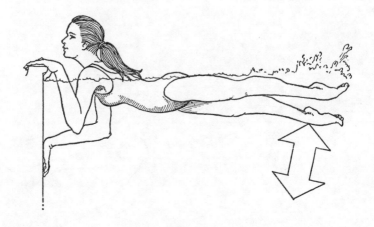

S-4
FLUTTER KICKING

Lying on your front, body straight and near the surface, legs extended. One hand on the edge of the pool or holding the gutter, palm facing down. Place the other hand, palm flat and fingers pointing *down*, against the poolside below the surface. (Pushing with this hand helps keep your legs afloat.)

Flutter-kicking action; one leg kicking downward as the other recovers upward.

Gentle, rhythmic, repetitive movement.

Allow a slight bend at the knee and at the hip.

Back flutter kicking can also be done. Start with your back to the poolside, body straight and near the surface, legs outstretched. Hold the side of the pool in either of two ways—arms outstretched, grasp deck or gutter *or* arms bent, elbows in front, reach over your shoulders, and grasp the deck or gutter with your hands (palms facing down). Use the method for holding onto the side of the pool that proves most comfortable for you.

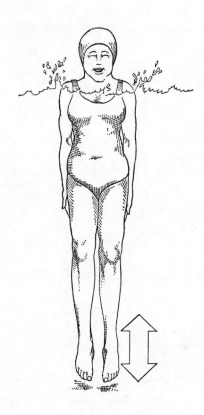

S-5
TOE BOUNCING

Standing.

Bounce up and down gently, extending the ankles and staying up on the toes.

Repetitions.

Stay erect, no bending at the knees or the hips.

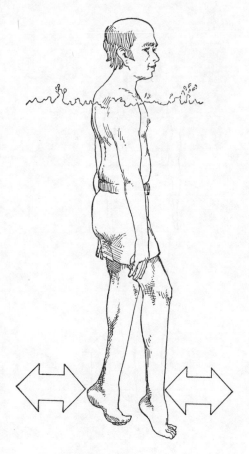

S-6
SPLIT BOUNCING

Standing, one leg in front of the other, feet about fifteen inches apart.

Jump up and reverse leg position for landing. That is, right in front, then left in front.

Repetitions, alternating leg positions for *each* landing.

Legs should be bent at the knees as you land. Land gently on the balls of the feet, *not* flatfooted.

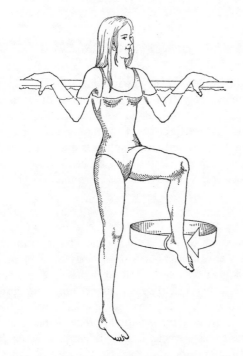

S-7
LOWER ROTATORS

Best done in ankle, knee, hip order. Holding the pool edge or gutter will help you keep balance for these three exercises.

Knee rotator: Standing on one leg, other leg lifted and bent at the knee *and* the hip so the thigh is parallel to the surface of water.

Slow, inward-sweeping circles with the lower leg. Rest. Repeat in the opposite direction. Rest. Repeat with the other leg.

Gentle, continuous, circular motion.

Large, slow circles, not small fast ones.

Ankle rotators and *hip rotators* are accomplished the same way, with rotation around the appropriate joint.

Swim Progression

If you're new to fitness and to swimming, you'll need a double measure of patience. If you're a poor swimmer or a nonswimmer, but think the water's for you, swimming lessons are a wise investment and a logical starting point. Once you master the basic strokes, you double your returns. Each session in the water brings improved skills *and* fitness. They build on one another.

As you progress, follow the FITTness Formula.

F—Frequency

Most pools do their best to cater to the fitness swimmer. Many recreation centers and fitness clubs open early to accommodate the early riser. Most also set aside at least some of the lanes for the noon-hour and after-work fitness swimmer. One recreation center near where I live has a half-price "night owl" session from 11:30 P.M. to 1:00 A.M. Shift workers greatly appreciate this extra service.

Keep the three-times-a-week maxim in mind. If your "water" is not easily accessible and there's travel time involved, you may want to mix your routine. Combine swimming with other activities. During-the-week swimming (if it's close to the office, for example) combined with some other activity on the weekend may be most appropriate. Or perhaps it's weekend swimming with the family and something else during the week. It's your choice. Don't get locked into one activity if that routine isn't right for you. It's the regularity, not the allegiance to one activity, that's important.

SWIMMING TARGET HEART RATES (TEN SECOND COUNT)

Age	25	30	35	40	45	50	55	60	65
"Fit Start"	21	21	20	19	18	17	17	16	16
"Keep Fit"	24	24	23	22	21	20	20	19	18

I—*Intensity*

If you're following the Chapter Two pulse-counting scheme, lower the target rates by one to two beats (in the ten-second count) as in the chart above. Use the "FIT START" or "KEEP FIT" level, whichever is appropriate for you *now*.

Swimming is primarily an arms, shoulders, and upper-body activity, placing greater demands on the heart. This lower pulse rate is more appropriate, helping to reduce the possibility of overexertion.

Remember the proper pulse-counting technique taught in Chapter Two. Most pools have a large deck clock with four colored hands set at fifteen-second intervals. A clock like this can help you get accurate counts. Ask the lifeguard if you don't see one around. It may be tucked away in a storeroom and only brought out when the swimming team practices.

T—*Time*

The beginning swimmer faces the same dilemma as the beginning runner. Fifteen minutes of continuous swimming may be difficult or impossible. If such is the case use interval training as suggested to the runners in Chapter Six. They have their telephone poles or city blocks for intervals. You'll have to stick to widths or lengths if you're in a pool. Swim a width or length, then rest, walking, flutter kicking, or doing some gentle water exercises until you feel ready to go again.

Follow this time-proven work-rest principle and soon you'll be "working" more and "resting" less. As fitness improves, you'll be swimming more widths or lengths before you need a rest. Later on, you'll be doing nonstop swimming at whatever speed proves best for you.

T—*Type*

Look outside swimming for ways to "work" in the water. Walking, running, skipping, hopping, bounding, and "paddling" are all legitimate forms of "work" and keep you busy as skill and fitness are improving. If you're not convinced of this, flutter kick (Exercise S-4) at a moderate pace for a minute or so, or run a width in chest-deep water with a high-knee action. Stop and take your pulse. This quickly shows that the nonswimmer can use the water to good advantage.

If you're a good swimmer, you can keep things interesting by broadening your swimming repertoire. Sidestroke, breaststroke, and elementary backstroke are the easy half of swimming's six strokes. The glide phase gives them their "resting stroke" label. Front and back crawl and butterfly are more difficult. They're harder to learn and require greater endurance in order to perform for any length of time. Beginners can include running, bounding, etc., with their swimming to give a good routine. Competent swimmers can mix resting strokes with the harder ones for an appropriate workout. Experiment and find what combination is right for you.

"Swimdown"—Cooldown

This remains an important part of any routine. Gentle activity—slower swimming, then walking in the shallow water—at the end of your session helps to ease your body back toward the resting state. Return to some of the water exercises. The upper rotators (S-1) are excellent to loosen up the shoulders and arms after a good swim.

Other Matters

Bathing Suits

Quick-drying nylon is the choice of competitive and fitness swimmers. One swim coach said you can expect eight to ten months' use from your suit at *two hours a day* in the water. That's about $.0150 an hour for men, $.0375 an hour for women at today's bathing-suit prices.

More expensive suits made of lycra (or half lycra and half nylon) are comfortable, stretchy, and fit skin tight. Many racers wear them for important competitions. For the recreational and fitness swimmer these suits offer no special advantages for the additional cost.

Goggles and Plugs

Eye infections from swimming are rare, so goggles aren't necessary as infection fighters. They do offer comfort, though, and can reduce or eliminate irritation and itchiness resulting from exposure to chemically treated water. If your eyes trouble you after swimming, goggles should be added to your swimming "wardrobe."

Two brands of goggles on the market are superior to all the others. They offer a tighter fit and work more effectively. Ask the competitive swimmers what they use. Experiment to see what brand best suits the contour around your eyes.

Eyes irritate, but ears can become infected. Public health codes ensure properly maintained pools, so ear infections aren't that common. But if you're susceptible to the problem, ear plugs are a wise purchase. Another precaution followed by some swim teams is swabbing the ears out with isopropyl alcohol after each workout. A small plastic bottle of alcohol and Q-tips kept with your towel and soap can make this a simple and regular routine. A physician friend offers, "Go easy with Q-tips, since they can irritate the external canal of the ear." He also suggests being gentle with your towel when cleaning the external ear. The best advice is to clean, but clean gently.

If chronic sinus trouble is a problem, nose clips are in order. They're shunned by competitive swimmers because they increase breathing resistance, but are wisely used by fitness swimmers who have or who develop this problem.

Injuries

Injuries often lead people *to* the pool; they rarely happen *in* it. But the long-distance types—like their cohorts in running and cycling—sometimes suffer from "overuse" injuries. Not surprisingly, the shoulder is the common problem area, and tendonitis is the normal villain. (Just like a runner's Achilles tendonitis.) This problem can afflict the fitness swimmer if his distance is considerable.

A minor case suggests a more leisurely routine until pain and discomfort subside. Ice massage (see Chapter Two) can help. When pain disappears, follow a *gradual* buildup to your former training distance. A more severe case may require rest, some ice massage and, perhaps, a visit to your doctor for specific advice. While you're recovering, you can still continue with legs-only swimming. Do your flutter kicking holding a styrofoam kickboard in front to rest your arms.

Another problem can visit breast strokers if they use a whipkick leg action instead of the old frog kick. This action, which has the knees close together and the toes turned dramatically outward, can bring soreness to the ligaments on the inside of the knees. Treatment includes ice massage and avoiding the stroke until recovered. If problems return, at worst you may have to delete this stroke from your repertoire or, at best, revert to the old frog kick.

Safety

The annual drowning rate is high. Most are accidents that could have been avoided. The Red Cross places a heavy emphasis on water-safety education. In or near the water, especially with children, take *no* chances. Watch your family and friends. Be your own lifeguard and use the "buddy" system. In ocean or lake swimming, don't overestimate your abilities or underestimate distance. Runners can stop and walk if they miscalculate. Swimmers face a more serious predicament. Follow the Red Cross dictum: "Be waterwise."

I've seen many sides of swimming, and it has brought me much joy. As a child I learned and played. As an athlete the water repaired injuries and soothed a flagging spirit, and as a teacher I was satisfied with enjoyment derived and skills improved.

But I think most of the silence and the motion. Runners and cyclists attune to their surroundings and flow with its changing personality. The pool swimmer doesn't see these daily differences so, in time, he may focus on the peace, the quiet, and the movement.

Lake or ocean swimming is a new adventure. A "swimmer" friend said to "runner" me, "It's not like a pool, you know. It's not always the same." I hadn't really thought about it before but, you know, he was right.

Wind and waves made for distant bobbing islands as we edged toward the neighbor's dock. Sun and clouds brought hues of blue and green to our water. I could leave running behind if allowed a swim in a warm, clear lake most days. Water, indeed, buoys the body. The action is graceful, relaxing, and pleasing. Even more, I found that the moving, the wind, the waves, and the distant bobbing islands buoyed my spirit.

President's Council on Physical Fitness and Sports. *Aqua Dynamics: Physical Conditioning Through Water Exercise*
Washington, D.C.: U. S. Government Printing Office (1977), 33 pp.

Shapiro, Sidney M. *Swim-nastics: Water Exercises for Better Health.*
Hollywood, Calif.: Creative Sports Books (1969), 65 pp.

CHAPTER NINE

Outdoors Unlimited

AEROBIC MISCELLANY

CROSS-COUNTRY SKIING

SNOWSHOEING

MOUNTAINEERING

ORIENTEERING

CANOEING AND KAYAKING

SURVIVAL

. . . Recently we opened a box from the country and were restored by the sharp smell of fir balsam and the flash of alderberry, as though we had received a transfusion from the great blood bank of New England. It is important that everyone feel strong and recognize the sources of his strength.

—E. B. White

THE TRADITIONAL city-fitness activities of walking, running, cycling, and swimming–not to omit skipping and indoor cycling–can prepare you for some exciting outdoor pursuits. In fact, thoughts of weekend or holiday outings may be the best motivators for weekday fitness maintenance. There's nothing like Monday-morning stiffness after Sunday's hike to remind you that once a week is not enough.

If you're turning to a new activity, you'll need some advice on what to get and how to start. I searched the bookstores and talked to the experts and compiled a very short list of reputable and popular "how to" books for beginners. The most-often recommended magazine in each field is also included. Check out local libraries, outdoor recreation equipment stores, and outdoor clubs for the "where to" information on your area.

Cross-country Skiing

Cross-country or nordic skiing is to be differentiated from downhill or alpine skiing. Cross-country is a great conditioner; downhill, with its short bursts of activity and forced rests in lineups and on lifts, is for recreation. You can cross-country ski yourself into shape, but you should be in shape for downhill. Notice all the new "pre-ski" exercise classes that accompanied the growth in alpine skiing. The big advantages of cross-country skiing include relatively inexpensive equipment and accessibility. Ski anywhere there's snow, regardless of terrain. For speed and excitement it's hard to beat downhill. But ski downhill for fun, not for fitness.

John Caldwell's book gives the basics on cross-country ski equipment and technique. *Nordic Skiing* magazine will keep you up to date.

Nordic Skiing (bimonthly, October to March)
P.O. Box 106
West Brattleboro, Vt. 05301

Caldwell, John. *The New Cross-Country Ski Book.*
New York: Bantam (1976)

Snowshoeing

Cross-country skiing is for those who slide comfortably into winter. Snowshoeing is for hikers who don't give in too easily. Gene Prater's book can help you start. With fewer participants and a less organized sport, snowshoeing does not yet have its own magazine. Both *Backpacker* (mentioned in Chapter Five) and *Nordic Skiing* periodically include some tips on snowshoeing.

Prater, Gene. *Snowshoeing.*
Seattle, Wash.: The Mountaineers (1974), 109 pp.

Mountaineering

Mountaineering, at the upper end of the walking-hiking continuum, offers great exhilarations to match its fierce demands. Attacking mountains with special climbing equipment is for the already fit (and fearless!). *Mountaineering: The Freedom of the Hills* is the accepted "textbook" of the sport. *Ascent* gives seventeen personal accounts by climbers who conquered their mountain. As a bonus it reviews nineteen books published on a wide range of mountaineering topics. *Summit,* one of the original magazines in the field, addresses itself to hiking and climbing.

Summit (ten issues yearly)
c/o Big Bear Lake, Calif. 92315

Ferber, Peggy (ed.). *Mountaineering: The Freedom of the Hills.*
Seattle, Wash.: The Mountaineers (1974), 478 pp.

Stack, Allan; Tejada-Flores, Lito; Stuart, Jim; and Roper, Steve, (eds.).
  Ascent: The Mountaineering Experience in Word and Image.
San Francisco: Sierra Club Books (1976), 128 pp.

Orienteering

Long a tool for survival, orienteering is gaining popularity in North America as a competitive activity. Likened to a car rally without the cars, participants negotiate their way through a course with map and compass. The smartest, not the swiftest, usually win.

It'll be some time before we rival the Scandinavians in this sport. National championships in Scandinavia attract upward of ten thousand *participants*. Imagine that? A traffic jam of people going somewhere to run!

Be Expert with Map and Compass, mentioned in Chapter Five, is your best introduction to this fascinating activity. Further assistance is available from the following:

RACING INFORMATION

Canadian Orienteering Federation
333 River Road
Vanier City, Ont. K1L 8B9
Canada

U.S. Orienteering Federation
317–933 North Kenmore Street
Arlington, Va. 22201

TEACHING AND TRAINING AIDS

American Orienteering Service
P.O. Box 547
La Porte, Ind. 43650

Canadian Orienteering Service
446 McNicolls Avenue
Willowdale, Ont. M2H 2E1

Canoeing and Kayaking

Just as swimmers find something special about being in the water, boaters long to be out *on* the water. Canoeing and kayaking bring the possibility of a wide range of water experience. At one end there's relaxing and peaceful lake or river canoeing; at the other end, the exhilaration of whitewater kayaking. Personal preference will determine what's right for you.

Canoe tripping can leave you with the same smug satisfaction the bike tripper feels. Canoeing is both back to nature and back to the basics. It's physically demanding and personally rewarding and allows you to visit territory accessible in no other way.

Canoeing and kayaking both have their "bible" of the sport and a regular magazine.

Canoe (bimonthly)
1999 Shepard Road
St. Paul, Minn. 55116

Down River (nine issues yearly, February to October)
World Publications
P.O. Box 366
Mountain View, Calif. 94040

Evans, Joy, and Anderson, Robert R. *Kayaking: The New Whitewater Sport for Everybody.*
Brattleboro, Vt.: The Stephen Greene Press (1975), 192 pp.

Riviere, Bill. *Pole, Paddle, and Portage: A Complete Guide to Canoeing.*
New York: Van Nostrand, Reinhold Company (1969), 259 pp.

Survival

Most outdoor books include safety precautions, first-aid procedures, and survival techniques. *Mountaineering Medicine* is a book to be read *and used.* It's a handy, little, forty-eight-page, take-along booklet that guides you in dealing with problems when they arise. A must for anyone wandering in the wilderness—summer or winter.

Darvill, Fred T., Jr., M.D. *Mountaineering Medicine: A Wilderness Medical Guide.*
Skagit Mountain Rescue Unit, Inc. (1975), 48 pp.
Mount Vernon, Washington

CHAPTER TEN

"I Feel Better"

THE REASONS

CORONARY HEART DISEASE

AGING

STRESS

LOW-BACK PAIN

WEIGHT CONTROL

"I FEEL BETTER"

To suggest that physical activity is an antidote to all the ills of modern society would be untruthful. But to pass lightly over its inherent benefits would be unwise. It's time now to consider these benefits. A fitness program must be built on a firm foundation. Part of this foundation is a proper understanding of what's to be gained.

Automation has long been taken for granted. Cars, escalators, elevators, and power—everything leaves little for us to wrestle with. Most jobs are sedentary ones. Physically demanding jobs are becoming increasingly mechanized. Hypokinesia (or insufficient movement) increasingly pervades our daily lives, and it's taking its toll. Drs. Hans Kraus and Wilhelm Raab, in their book *Hypokinetic Disease*, documented a wide range of diseases that appear to occur more often among sedentary people than among the more active.

Their list was a long one. Chronic fatigue, shortness of breath, overweight, digestive upsets, headache, backache, and anxiety states were on their list. Muscular weakness and musculoskeletal pain and injuries were included, as were high blood pressure, coronary artery disease, and "generalized, accelerated, degenerative" aging.

The reasons for activity, considered here, are discussed in no particular order, certainly not in order of importance, since that's very much a subjective thing. If anything, we move through the intangible and quite nebulous benefits to the practical, daily-experienced ones.

Coronary Heart Disease

Coronary heart disease (CHD), sometimes called the disease of prosperity or the disease of affluence, is a massive problem in North America. It's the single greatest cause of death and disability in men over thirty-five. More than a million and a half heart attacks occur in North America each year. Almost half of the victims die immediately or within one year. Of the survivors, 40 to 60 per cent can anticipate full recovery. The remainder can expect continued impairment varying from mild to extensive.

Science has identified a number of factors that increase the risk of heart disease. Those we can do something about include high-fat/high-cholesterol diets, cigarette smoking, high blood pressure, excessive weight, physical inactivity, and anxiety (how we respond to stress).

The role of physical activity in the prevention of coronary heart disease has been under exploration for some time. Early studies examined the incidence of heart attacks in those pursuing physically active occupations compared to those in less active jobs. Be it mail carriers vs. mail sorters, bus conductors vs. drivers, railroad yard workers vs. clerks, or longshoremen vs. their deskbound cohorts, the results were the same. Those in the more physically active jobs had a lower risk of an initial heart attack, had a better chance of survival if an attack did occur, and held greater prospects for full recovery.

Additional studies have considered the protective mechanism of appropriate leisuretime activities. One of the biggest and best-known studies examined the leisuretime habits of seventeen thousand British civil servants who held sedentary jobs. Those who reported *regular* moderate to vigorous physical activity of sufficient duration had about one third the incidence of coronary disease as those whose recreational activities were of a sedentary nature. Activities found appropriate included brisk walking, swimming, digging in the garden, and other heavy work. Those involved in very light exercise appeared to have no greater immunity than the nonexercisers.

Coronary heart disease is a general term applied to the various forms of heart disease that are caused by a narrowing or a blockage of the coronary arteries. Coronary arteries surround the heart and carry the blood (and oxygen) to the heart muscle so it can pump endlessly to keep us working, playing, eating, and sleeping. CHD develops slowly over a period of many years. As the disease progresses, cholesterol and other fatty materials become embedded in the inner walls of the arteries. In time, these deposits accumulate and grow in size so these channels, through which the blood must flow, narrow and roughen. Ultimately, total blockage may result from a blood clot catching in a fat-laden, already narrowed artery.

This blockage deprives the heart of the oxygen it needs to do its job. In some cases, sudden death results. Other heart-attack victims survive but face the prospect of rehabilitation toward partial or complete recovery.

Exercise reduces the risk of CHD both directly and indirectly. Indirectly, it has a positive moderating influence on some of the other coronary risk factors. Mild reductions in blood pressure can be achieved through regular exercise of the appropriate type. Weight control is aided by regular activity.

More directly, scientists suggest a number of ways that sufficient fitness manifests itself in heart-attack protection. Emergencies, sudden demands, and unaccustomed overexertion require larger than normal supplies of oxygen to the heart in order for it to complete its task. It is these short, demanding bursts of activity that can be dangerous to the very untrained heart. The trained heart completes its task more comfortably and efficiently, thus facing a lower risk of insufficient oxygen, which can lead to irregular heart beats and, in some cases, to heart failure. Regular moderate activity prepares the heart for occasional supreme efforts.

Some authorities suggest that an important change occurs in the heart region itself, which is paramount in the protective mechanism. Their contention is that stamina training develops additional coronary arteries. These new pathways provide alternative routes for the blood (and oxygen) if an artery becomes blocked. More pathways help avert a heart attack.

All the evidence is not in, but it's apparent that prevention is the key, and exercise can help. A joint working party of the Royal College of Physicians of London and the British Cardiac Society stated:

> We consider that the present size of the CHD problem in this country and the small effect of medical and surgical treatment on the mortality rate from CHD justify attempts to prevent the disease we cannot cure.

Furthermore, Dr. Kavanaugh, in *Heart Attack? Counter Attack!* says:

> . . . the evidence to date is increasingly compelling, and ten years from now it may be complete. But that may be ten years too late for some!

Aging

Advancing age brings changes in our physical characteristics—changes that are slow, progressive, and barely perceptible. Quite naturally, we lose our endurance, our strength, and the elasticity in our muscles. Formerly simple tasks can be more burdensome. One gets winded more easily, recovers more slowly, and fatigue may linger. Stiffness unknown in our youth can plague us after a day's work in the garden. These very tangible physical aspects of aging are hastened by an inactive lifestyle but slowed if one exercises as a way of life. Unfortunately, there's no guarantee that one will live longer if more active, but one can certainly *live younger longer*.

In North America, advancing age is often accepted graciously, and "retirement" at sixty-five is the order of the day. These facts make it difficult for us to imagine cultures where "retirement" is not in the dictionary, where "middle age" stretches into the eighties, and where those over a hundred years of age assume important duties and contribute to the economy of their communities. But these cultures do exist.

The most famous of them are Vilcabamba in the mountains of Ecuador, the land of Hunza in the Karakoram Range in Kashmir, and Abkhazia in the South of the Soviet Union. They share some common traits, ones we'd be wise to take note of and ponder. Their diets, active lifestyles, lack of stress, no retirement policy, and outlook on aging reflect a way of life quite unlike our own.

Their mountainous terrain means that pastureland is scarce, making animal husbandry nearly impossible. For this reason, fats of animal origin constitute a very small portion of most diets. Cholesterol levels of many centenarians is reportedly less than half the amount looked upon as normal for North Americans aged fifty to sixty.

The aged of all three cultures share a great deal of physical activity. Farming is a way of life from childhood to death. Dealing with the mountainous terrain on a daily basis ensures high levels of fitness.

Emotional stress is not a big factor in their lives, and a feeling of usefulness pervades one's entire lifetime. But the most intriguing aspect is their attitude toward getting old. When asked, the "youth" of Abkhazia said they expected to live beyond one hundred years. It's very much a psychological thing. Whereas we may accept early aging, they are incapable of comprehending that sixty-five could be "old."

Recent reports suggest that early studies may have exaggerated the ages of these people, and they may have seemed an older population merely because many of the young people moved away. However, scientists conducting the early studies had suggested it was the fitness level of many of the elderly more than their extreme age that most impressed them.

Needless to say, for most of us, catching a plane to Ecuador is out of the question. But their secrets to success are lifestyle things, and these we can do something about, right here at home. To a great extent, we control our own fates. We can change our diets, activity patterns, ways of handling stress, and our outlooks on life and living.

Perhaps, in years to come, as prudent lifestyles become increasingly common, more of us will personally understand what Temur Tarba, resident of Abkhazia, USSR, meant when he said:

> It is best to be a youth, but I have good health, feel well, have wonderful children, and I enjoy myself greatly now. . . . Every day is a gift when you are over a hundred.

Stress

Some people are luckier than others. The placid, smiling, and relaxed types glide, float, and move along comfortably. Life's little irritations don't get them down. For others, life is more tumultuous. They "mobilize" and prepare for action more often. Irritating phone calls, meetings that lead nowhere, and traffic jams take their toll. Life's little irritations become big ones.

Some very basic physical changes occur as one "prepares for action," so to speak. Adrenalin pours into the system, muscles tense, breathing and heart rate speed up, and blood pressure rises. These reactions known collectively as the fight-or-flight response, were important in primitive times when movement was crucial to survival. Man did, in fact, fight or flee. Our innate fight-or-flight response is still with us but, in most cases, we are denied the opportunity of fighting or running.

Instead of fighting or running, we are usually forced to sit and fume. This repeated elicitation of the fight-or-flight response, with its attendant transient elevations in blood pressure, can lead to a permanent state of hypertension. This in turn can contribute to the development of coronary heart disease.

The obvious first step is to glide and float more often—mobilize for action less often. Conscious and constant practice may be necessary for some as they develop a new, more relaxed attitude toward life. Note the increased popularity of yoga, Transcendental Meditation, and other stress-reduction techniques to help in this quest. (Herbert Benson, in *The Relaxation Response*, discusses the fascinating mechanisms of stress and relaxation. He details a simple, self-taught relaxation technique. The book sells for less than ten dollars and is valuable reading for anyone considering TM—*before* signing up.)

Relaxation is important. Our other alternative—flight—can still play a part. We can't always flee exactly when we want to, but we *can* flee daily. Dr. Hans Selye, the world's foremost researcher on the effects of stress, suggests that training in a sensible exercise program sets up a "cross resistance" against emotional stress.

Similarly, Chapter 18 of *Life and Health* states:

> Deliberate and appropriate exercise, then, enables modern man to release psychological tension and achieve physical relaxation.

Psychiatrist Thaddeus Kostrubala, in *The Joy of Running*, talks of using running in the treatment of patients with anxiety, depression, and even schizophrenia. "Running therapy" brought improvements to some who had not responded to any of the other, more traditional forms of therapy.

Jerome Drayton, Canadian marathoner, sixth in the Montreal Olympics, suggests that running is "active meditation." Runners know what he means. We know how well it works. I, for one, have to get out and move for a while—just about every day. It's not something I consciously think about. My body usually tells me when it's time to go. On some days I need it more than on others. It takes time before you understand how well this fleeing works, but it remains a strong draw once experienced.

Low-back Pain

Low-back pain, like heart disease, has reached monumental proportions. Workdays lost and the annual compensation bill for back injuries in the workplace are alarming. Dr. Kraus suggests that fully 80 per cent of low-back-pain cases result from *underexercise*. In his opinion, "garden variety" low-back pain is one of the major ailments of our mechanized society.

Low-back pain has a twofold origin. First, repeated tensing of muscles, as occurs when the fight-or-flight response is elicited, can result in a loss in muscle length. Shortened back muscles are more susceptible to overstretching and injury.

Second, physical inactivity harbors muscle weakness and inflexibility. The occupational sitting position allows the stomach muscles to relax and weaken over time. As suggested in Chapter Three, these muscles are meant to work with the muscles in the back, helping support the spine, keeping it erect, and maintaining proper posture. Without the stomach muscles playing their part, a forward tilt of the pelvis and curvature of the lower spine can result. Excess weight in the stomach area accentuates the problem, bringing an even more pronounced forward tilt of the pelvis. In this case, inflexible back muscles, weak stomach muscles, and excess weight create a more vulnerable target for back pains and strains.

The lower back can only act effectively as the foundation for movement if it is conditioned and well cared for. The vertebrae of the spine are separated by shock-absorbing pads called discs. If these are positioned properly and weight bearing is distributed over their entire surface they can absorb large compression forces. However, when the spine is in an unnatural position (through poor posture or an incorrect lifting position, for example), the discs are subject to great strain since the forces act on only a small portion of their overall surface. The potential for problems increases with age, since discs tend to lose their water content becoming less resilient.

If muscles don't work efficiently and they fail to keep the spine within its normal range of movement, the ligaments (which are straplike lengths of fibrous tissue tying the vertebrae together) are stretched and may be strained. Ligaments are designed to prevent excessive movement at the joints of the spine. Ligaments can be injured when the strain is too great (for example, lifting an overly heavy object) or maintained too long (for example, working in a low-ceiling basement). Strong muscles prevent excessive movement of the ligaments which, in turn, help protect the vertebrae of the spine and the discs that separate them.

Strong muscles do protect the spine, but while the muscles act as "protectors" for others, they are not immune to injury themselves. Sudden or unexpected overloading can stretch the muscles beyond the length to which they are accustomed and cause muscle strains and tears. Similarly, holding an extreme position for a long period of time can strain a fatigued muscle. Supple muscles can exert their forces comfortably over a wider range and thus carry out their job as "protectors" more effectively.

This job as "protector" may, in fact, depend as much on the inherent suppleness of the muscle as it does on its strength. Ligaments and tendons have little elasticity, so to ensure that they are not overstretched the muscle is the one that must be able to "give."

This "give" or suppleness of the muscle is a tricky thing. To be technically correct, one must speak of the elasticity of the *connective tissue*. As the name implies, this tissue connects the muscle to the tendon, which in turn attaches to the bone. Individual muscle fibers, which are grouped into bundles and surrounded by connective tissue to make up a muscle, have no ability to stretch. The stretch occurs at the end of the bundles, where the connective tissue joins the tendon. Since the body of the muscle itself, along with ligaments and tendons, has little elasticity, increased suppleness results as the connective tissue near the tendon becomes more pliable.

A certain amount of activity is necessary merely to *maintain* a given range of movement. Restriction of movement is a progressive process, and connective tissue tends to shorten if it is not taken through its full range *regularly*. Perhaps this is why the inactive become even less inclined and less capable of activity later in life.

Regular and progressive stretching can first increase and then help maintain a wide range of movement in the various muscles and joint regions. Overstretching is then less likely to occur. Specific strengthening exercises ensure adequate muscle strength, thus helping minimize the strain on ligaments, tendons, vertebrae, and discs. Occupational and recreational injuries and accidents can be reduced if appropriate exercise is pursued on a regular basis.

Gardening provides an opportunity for the muscles to stretch and remain elastic. Heavy gardening and lifting call the stomach muscles into action, helping them maintain a certain degree of strength. *Appropriate* yoga exercises are excellent means of maintaining suppleness. At the more advanced levels, yoga also helps develop strength if enough antigravity exercises are included. A daily exercise routine as outlined in Chapter Three achieves the same end. A regular program makes Monday-morning stiffness a thing of the past. A regular program allows you to attack other physical tasks with greater enthusiasm, less risk of injury, and less residual soreness.

Weight Control

Exercise, to this point, has been considered within a framework of what it can do—how it can help. To keep the exercise-and-weight-control issue straight, it is best considered in the light of what exercise *can't* do. What it can't do—as the *sole* vehicle for weight *loss*—is achieve success in the time span that most people are willing to endure.

Consider these facts. One pound equals 3,500 calories. Your average piece of strawberry shortcake is about 400 calories. To "burn off" the shortcake requires 1¼ hours of walking (at 3 mph pace), 50 minutes of cycling (at 10 mph), or 35 minutes of swimming or running. A mile run, for example, consumes only about 100 calories. It's plain to see that if you intend to lose a significant amount of weight through increased activity alone, you must also plan to be very busy and extremely tired.

It is now well recognized that the most effective approach to weight loss is increased physical activity in combination with dietary change. The two together are more successful than either pursued alone. Dietary change should consist of a reduction of the total number of calories consumed per day and a move to reduce or eliminate the intake of nonnutritious foods (that is, those high in fats and sugars). The key to long-term success is *a change in eating habits* so that unwanted pounds *stay off*. Fad diets that offer quick success are usually followed by a return of the weight lost and a search for the next "newest, surest way to lose weight forever." As

weight loss progresses, increased physical activity, along with helping to burn off calories, helps improve strength and muscle tone so
that one doesn't appear a "saggy" lighter person but as one whose
body really belongs to him.

While a reduction in food intake is crucial to weight loss, it must
be remembered that a well-balanced, healthful diet is *equally* important. Protein is necessary to build and maintain body tissue.
Minerals (inorganic substances) are vital to several body functions.
For example, calcium, which is plentiful in milk and milk products,
provides most of the structure of bones and teeth. Iron, found in
meat and meat alternatives, affects the oxygen-carrying ability of
the blood. Vitamins are special chemicals required in small
amounts to act as catalysts for important bodily reactions. Carbohy-
drates and fats supply calories (energy) for daily activity. A well-
balanced diet brings these important nutrients.

Problems arise when food intake is in excess of that required for
energy expenditure. This intake-output imbalance in the "calorie
bank" results in the excess being stored as fat throughout the body.
This weight gain is usually a slow, insidious process brought on by
two main factors.

The first is a gradual reduction in the body's metabolic rate with
advancing age. As the metabolic rate slows, the body's daily energy
requirements decrease (very slowly and gradually, remember).
This means that maintaining the same food intake and activity level
results in a weight gain—a most depressing prospect. The secret
lies in reducing food intake or increasing activity level (or both) as
"old age" approaches. For those inactive in their youth, a change in
both diet and exercise level is a wise solution (like fewer doughnuts
and more walking). If you're regularly active, you'd best address
the issue with a maintenance of activity level while reducing food
intake.

Second, a very small imbalance in the "calorie bank" can wreak
havoc over time. A daily hundred-calorie excess means creeping
obesity—a ten-pound weight gain in one year. Toast and jam fans,
grabbing that extra piece at breakfast or snacking before bed, are
looking at more than one hundred calories per piece. This presents
no problem if it's part of daily requirements and the bank is balanced. But if it's bonus calories, a year of toast and jam converts to
a hefty weight gain.

The secret is *moderation.* The proper combination of food intake and daily activity can comfortably ensure a proper body weight with advancing age. And sustaining a normal or "ideal" body weight is important for personal health maintenance. Those markedly overweight are at greater risk of developing heart disease because of the increased likelihood of high blood pressure, elevated blood cholesterol, and diabetes.

"I Feel Better"

"Feeling better" is the strongest of the practical motivators. A desire for weight loss spurs some to action. A need to curb low-back pain gets others going. But these are "starter" motivators and they're only enough to keep most people going for a short period of time—a few days to a few weeks. A more tangible motivator is the "feeling better" that comes with appropriate, sensible activity. Exercise proves to be a powerful energy source. It works wonders at recharging human batteries.

Some very basic changes occur as fitness improves, and it is these changes that lead to the "feeling better" feeling. The heart and lungs become more efficient, making a more powerful system for transporting oxygen. The muscles become more adept at picking up oxygen as the heart pumps it to them. In effect, the maximum capacity of the system increases. All daily tasks are then carried out at a lower percentage of that maximum capacity. It's a strange paradox. By working the body moderately hard for short periods of time on a regular basis, it doesn't have to work as hard the rest of the time. This means less fatigue from each task, less tiredness at day's end, and bonus energy for other activities.

I'm not about to suggest what form this "feeling better" might take in your life. In fact, I have absolutely no way of knowing. But I do know that it comes in many guises and is most important to those who persist long enough to experience it.

One says, "Now I can throw a ball around with my kids and not get tired." A second noticed an improvement in his golf swing a few weeks after he started his exercises. A third said he used to stop and rest at the top of the steep path between his garage and house. After a few weeks of cycling he said, "On Saturday, I climbed the stairs with my two-year-old daughter in one arm, a bag of potatoes in the other. I got into the house before it dawned on me I had climbed the stairs and wasn't the least bit out of breath."

A most heartful description of "feeling better" came from a participant in one of our exercise classes. In response to a questionnaire asking what value she found in the class she attended, she replied:

> It is significant. I arrive a lazy, tired, and rheumatically cranky middle-aged lady, and I leave full of vitality and well-being toward the world in general. I have not felt so happy for a long time. This overflows into my working life, where—I do not need to detail—one encounters so many irritants. Of course, I still succumb to them. . . . But I find I am better able to cope. I sincerely mean this.
>
> I am less winded.
>
> I think I look better, and to one who has reached face-lift time, this is important.
>
> There is the satisfaction of seeing neglected limbs becoming . . . very, very gradually in my case . . . supple. I have a long way to go.
>
> I consider Yogaerobics* ideal for me. It is interesting to observe that even after running almost a mile, one's limbs are very much out of condition when used for a different type of movement. Also, one complements the active approach with the contemplative.
>
> One has the opportunity of observing the insidious result of not using one's body effectively over the years.

So these are some of the reasons—the motivations for physical activity. Some help you start, others keep you going. Some will be important to you, others you'll hardly consider. These motivators can get you to that strange point in time when you need no justification for what you're doing—when you're active because you want to be, because it feels good and, perhaps, because now you really can't go without it. And if you're lucky enough to reach this stage, you've come upon the most powerful motivator of all.

* A yoga and running class.

Benson, Herbert, M.D. *The Relaxation Response.* New York: Avon (1976), 222 pp.

Selye, Hans, M.D. *The Stress of Life*.
New York: McGraw-Hill (1956), 324 pp.

———. *Stress Without Distress*.
Philadelphia: J. B. Lippincott Company (1974), 150 pp.

CHAPTER ELEVEN
The End . . . the Beginning

WELL, IT's just about the end for me. I've done my part—done all that I can do. And now, perhaps, a beginning for you.

George Sheehan once wrote of his beginning,

> At the age of reason, I was placed on a train, the shades drawn, my life's course and destination already determined. At the age of forty-five, I pulled the emergency cord and ran out into the world. It was a decision that meant no less than a new life, a new course, a new destination. I was born again in my forty-fifth year.

This book has been largely about beginning—about starting and persisting—the time when the sacrifices seem great while the immediate rewards are small. Many start with fine intentions but don't last. You need all the help you can get in this early, hard part. It's a formidable foe and it wins its share of battles. The advice here offered was to increase the odds in your favor. In summary, lest you forget:

Revisit Chapter Two. Plan wisely. Consider the activities of Chapters Four through Nine in the light of Chapter Two's planning advice. Start with the health checklist and see your physician if PAR-Q suggests it. Heed the precautions and follow the FITTness Formula. Return to the Principles for Persisting in weaker moments.

Spend time with Chapter Three. Suppleness and strength—important components of fitness—are often passed over lightly. They deserve serious attention.

Choose your activity with the utmost care. "Nonmovers" should give serious thought to all possible alternatives before settling on an indoor-equipment routine (for the reasons mentioned in Chapter Four). Remember that boredom is self-inflicted. Fight ruts. Look for variety. Change your activity if things aren't going well.

That's my final sally of advice. The rest is up to you.

But along with all this advice, I've tried for something more. My professional and practical selves dealt with the advice, the "ways and means," and it was not so difficult, really—it's all so straight-forward and tangible. But writing of the "joys and insights" that come after fitness is achieved has been a fascinating and more difficult struggle. I relied heavily on the words of others to help build my case, but even then I reach this point with some uncertainty. Did these words suitably convey the "feeling" of it all?

I take solace in knowing that others also struggle. Michael Murphy, in *Golf in the Kingdom,* tried to explain what his friend Shivas Irons felt and what it was he hoped for. Murphy wrote:

> . . . When I come to putting it down on paper I have a feeling that I am forcing his vision; that no matter how I state the goal he would set, there is something left over that words will always leave out.

Perhaps we shouldn't worry that our words may fall short of the mark. Joe Henderson writes of running:

> The artistic satisfaction we feel isn't transferable. It can't be passed along to nonrunners—or even other runners, it's nearly impossible to put into words, it can hardly be re-membered. The excitement and satisfaction reside in the run itself.

I also recognize that what I feel—what I derive from my activity—is not necessarily what you will feel. But I had to dwell on these thoughts for a while, however uncontainable and individual they may be. To talk only of the "ways and means"—of the starting and persisting—would be a grave injustice.

I admitted much earlier to being an habitual addicted "mover." Addiction is not a word that one throws around lightly, and I really meant it. But I'm not so different. Many of us are compelled to daily moving and can only be thankful it's good for us. I, for one, would surely carry on even if it weren't.

So this addiction has been with many of us for some time, but only recently has it been studied, formalized, and documented. William Glasser did this well in *Positive Addiction,* setting out certain characteristics of activities that made them amenable to positive addiction (PA). The requirements were:

- An activity you *choose* to do, either physical or mental.

- A belief that it has value for you and of enough worth to put an hour a day into.

- Something you are, or can become, proficient in, and of enough intrinsic value so you'll stick to it long enough to reach the PA state (which, in many cases, may take up to a year).

Glasser calls them positive addictions because "they strengthen us and make our lives more satisfying." He says:

> The beautiful part of positive addiction is that whatever it is we ordinarily don't need it. It is an extra that we choose to do. No one needs to run by himself for an hour at six in the morning, rain or shine, but if we do it, who would care about it except ourselves?

He talked at length of running, yoga, and TM, and evaluated their addictive powers. The "addicted" who responded to his questionnaire suggested that their addictive activity was accompanied by a trancelike mental state and that the activity was pleasurable, relaxing, and felt very good. Many, who by their questionnaire responses were obviously addicted, had great difficulty in describing exactly what their activity meant to them.

A young girl I once tested and counseled, struggled this same way trying to express her feelings. Her favorite sports included ice skating, swimming, and roller skating. The swimming and ice skating she preferred in the company of friends. She liked roller skating best but found it most satisfying when pursued alone. This often meant an afternoon session at a nearby arena. But whenever possible she went to the top of a hill that housed a covered reservoir, swept a path, and skated alone. She didn't say much but it was easy to sense that it was more than just a physical thing for her. That lonely reservoir offered something the arena did not have.

Juha Vaatainen, a Finnish distance runner, said quite simply:

> I enjoy the applause. But I realize this is only temporary. I live each day at a time and seek only my own pleasure. I long to discover new faces every day. But I also like solitude. Running for me is a very lonely affair. I very often train alone.
>
> I don't like to go around a track. Outside of competition I never do it. Actually stadiums were built for spectators, not for runners. We have nature and that's much better.

So whether it's the aloneness, nature, or something quite different that brings you your "feelings," it really doesn't matter. The intriguing fact remains that each person derives something unique from his activity. In addition, each individual comes to know what it means to him in a place and at a time also uniquely his own.

My realization came nine years ago. I was one month and four thousand miles away from the most important athletic competition of my life. It wasn't eighty degrees and sunny and there weren't thousands of people watching. I was running alone on a dirt road in the woods. It was drizzling, the trees were fragrant, I felt strong, and my legs were fresh.

I thought back to that day a month ago and it seemed, somehow, less powerful or significant. With the simplicity of this day came the understanding that running here all alone meant just as much to me as that competition did. Then I really knew that the moving's the thing and, if there's something that's to be a brief part of every day that awaits me, I know of nothing finer.